Y0-DDS-940

This publication is designed to provide authoritative information in regard
to the subject matter covered. Many of the product designations are clarified
by trademarks. While every precaution has been taken in the preparation of
this book, the author assumes no responsibility for errors or omissions, or
damages resulting from the use of information contained herein.

This book is available at special quantity discounts.

For additional information, please contact our support team:

https://CompletelyKeto.com/support

1-866-FOR-KETO

2019051410ALSPP

Table of Contents

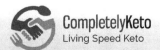

Disclaimer

Welcome! We're excited to have you with us on this journey. All of the information provided in the book and on the website located at https://completelyketo.com is intended solely for general information and should NOT be relied upon for any particular diagnosis, treatment, or care. This book is not a substitute for medical advice. The book and website are only for general informational purposes.

The information contained in this book is not a substitute for medical advice or treatment, and the author strongly encourages patients and their families to consult with qualified medical professionals for treatment and related advice on individual cases.

Decisions relating to the prevention, detection, and treatment of all health issues should be made only after discussing the risks and benefits with your health care provider, as well as considering your personal medical history, your current situation and your future health risks and concerns. If you are pregnant, nursing, diabetic, on medication, have a medical condition, or are beginning a health or weight control program, consult your physician before using products or services discussed in this book and before making any other dietary changes. This diet is not recommended or supported for those under the age of eighteen. By using this book, you represent that you are at least eighteen (18) years old and a United States resident.

The author cannot guarantee that the information in this book is safe and proper for every reader. For this reason, this book is offered without warranties or guarantees of any kind, expressed or implied, and the author disclaims any liability, loss, or damage caused by the contents thereof, either directly or consequentially. The U.S. Food and Drug Administration or any other government regulatory body has not evaluated the statements made in this book. Products, services, and methods discussed in this book are not intended to diagnose, treat, cure, or prevent any disease.

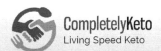

CompletelyKeto
Living Speed Keto

Chapter 1

Introduction

Many of you have already completed a few rounds of Speed Keto and are ready for a new menu plan while others reading this will be brand new to the ketogenic lifestyle. You should really start with our Speed Keto program and use Living Speed Keto as a follow up.

If you've tried to lose weight unsuccessfully in the past this is the eating program that will change your life.

What's it all about?

Living Speed Keto is a 31 day, month-long program.

Why you should choose a Ketogenic meal plan

A ketogenic eating plan purposefully limits the amount of carbohydrates consumed while allowing for the consumption of moderate amounts of protein and a higher consumption of fats. This allows the liver to break down stored body fat (adipose) into a source of energy the body can easily use called ketone bodies. As ketone levels become higher the body moves into a state we call ketosis where stored body fat is being burned as the main source of fuel.

Simply stated, the goal of a ketogenic diet is to stay in ketosis. The Living Speed Keto plan includes delicious recipes, tailor-made to keep you in ketosis and burning fat.

Short term and long term intermittent fasting

While I recommend intermittent fasting, it is optional during your month of Living Speed Keto. Choosing to fast will speed up your weight loss. It is exactly as it sounds; periods of eating nothing in between periods of consuming food. There are two types of intermittent fasting employed:

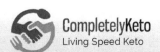
CompletelyKeto
Living Speed Keto

- Short Term: less than 24 hours
- Long Term: more than 24 hours

Fasting speeds up weight loss, provides rest for stressed body organs and promotes healing. While you do abstain from eating meals during fasting periods you will always be allowed to drink water. In addition, bulletproof coffee and sugar-free electrolyte drinks are all allowed. Organic chicken broth can also be taken during the day as desired.

If you choose to fast during this month, my goal is to make this as easy for you as possible. We've already led thousands of people through fasts, and most are able to make it through fine. In fact, the number one response we hear is: "I could have gone on longer."

BUT ... if you feel ill, tired, or just not 100% (for any reason) you should stop fasting and eat immediately. I also recommend that everyone consult with a physician before starting this process.

The 31 day menu plan shows the fasting periods clearly. If you decide to opt out of fasting simply choose recipes from our breakfast, lunch or dinner selections in the recipe section of this book.

OMAD (one meal a day)

A short term 23-hour fast, with a one hour window for eating a single meal (24 hours altogether),is also referred to as one meal a day or OMAD. The Living Speed Keto menu plan includes four OMAD days during the second and fourth weeks of the month-long program. Once again please note that fasting during this month is entirely optional.

If you do opt into some or all of the fasting periods you will likely find eating one meal a day to be fairly easy once you get used to it. Most people doing OMAD choose to skip breakfast and usually work through lunch. For those at home finding activities away from the house on OMAD days helps too.

The one meal a day you are allowed to eat (consumed during a one hour period) is especially delicious as anticipation and ultimately appreciation intensifies along with hunger.

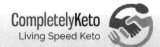

CompletelyKeto
Living Speed Keto

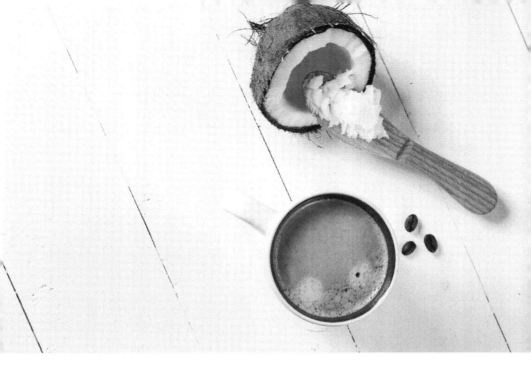

Bulletproof Coffee — What is it?

We allow fat fortified Bulletproof Coffee every morning which will satisfy the appetite and help curb cravings throughout the morning and into the afternoon.

Coffee is a healthy drink that boosts metabolism, so don't shy away from including it in your diet. We do urge you to select certified organic coffee when making a purchase. Two teaspoons of heavy cream are allowed in a cup of coffee. However, watch the number of cups consumed because we want you to minimize dairy consumption during the 31 day program.

To make Bulletproof Coffee you will be adding MCT Oil or MCT Oil Powder to your morning cup of coffee, with the addition of heavy cream being optional. The added fat means added fuel. When you are doing OMAD or other forms of fasting, the energy boost from Bulletproof Coffee really helps curb the appetite. It also tastes great!

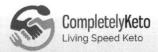

CompletelyKeto
Living Speed Keto

MCT Oil

MCT Oil stands for medium-chain triglyceride oil. This form of fat is immediately accessible as an energy source for your body. It doesn't need a lot of processing in the liver. Your brain loves medium chain triglycerides and gobbles them up! Adding this oil to your coffee in the morning helps clear up a foggy brain and gives you immediate energy for tackling a busy day.

It also supports ketosis which is just what you want on Living Speed Keto. You will find quite a few different brands of MCT oils out there but they are not all equal. It really matters what the MCT oil is made from. Most MCT oil comes from coconut oil. Cheaper varieties are often manufactured using too much caproic acid which has a throat burning sensation. Others use lauric acid which does not convert to ketones.

Completely Keto MCT oil powder is a delicious and wonderful way to get your MCT oils.

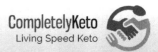

Chapter 2

"NO" Food

Food restrictions during 31 days of Living Speed Keto ...

Foods you might find on a regular ketogenic diet may not appear in the list of allowed foods for the Speed Keto and Living Speed Keto programs I've designed. My team and I have chosen foods and formulated a 31 day plan that alternates eating delicious food with different types of fasting. These programs are formulated to maximize weight loss.

Sometimes people will plateau in terms of their weight loss goals, even when eating the regular Keto diet and watching their macro ratios. A number of factors can contribute to a weight loss stall and switching to a Speed Keto diet for 31 days often helps break the plateau and re-start the bathroom scales on that downward trend.

If you are dealing with a medical condition such as metabolic syndrome, PCOS or Type 2 diabetes you are likely insulin resistant. This means you may have trouble getting into ketosis, especially at the beginning of a ketogenic diet. The Speed Keto Diet and Living Speed Keto program will help your body make the transition from being a glucose burning furnace into one that thrives on ketones.

No to nuts ...

We don't include nuts on Speed Keto or Living Speed Keto for one simple reason; nuts are really easy to over-consume and they are inflammatory to many people. Products made with nuts, like nut butters and nut flours are even more calorie-dense. It takes 90 almonds to make a single cup of almond flour! Give nuts, nut butters and flours a break for 31 days of Living Speed Keto and see what a difference this can make.

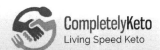

CompletelyKeto
Living Speed Keto

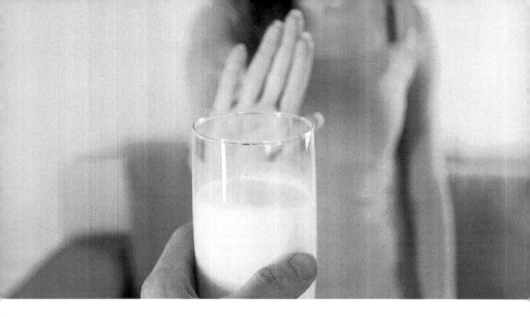

No to seeds too!

Seeds are also not included. A simple sprinkle to garnish that stir-fry also adds carbs to your daily count. When working to keep this count as low as possible, an extra sprinkle of sesame seeds doesn't make good sense.

Psyllium and flax seeds are often used as ways to include fiber in a ketogenic diet. The thinking behind this strategy is these seeds will bulk up the stool and prevent constipation. However, a study to investigate the effect of reducing dietary fiber on patients with idiopathic constipation was carried out between 2008 and 2010. The study concluded: "Idiopathic constipation and its associated symptoms can be effectively reduced by stopping or even lowering the intake of dietary fiber."[1]

Meat contains fiber as well as plants, especially in the connective tissues. When on the Living Speed Keto eating plan, you should expect the volume of stool to be less but this is natural given the restriction of carbohydrates.

---

1 Kok-Sun Ho, Charmaine You Mei Tan, Muhd Ashik Mohd Daud, Francis Seow-Choen. Stopping or reducing dietary fiber intake reduces constipation and its associated symptoms. World Journal of Gastroenterology, September 7, 2012, Volume 18, Issue 33 2012 September 7; 18(33): 4593-4596ISSN 1007-9327 (print) ISSN 2219-2840 (online) https://www.ncbi.nlm.nih.gov/pmc/articles/PMC3435786/pdf/WJG-18-4593.pdf

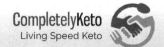

CompletelyKeto
Living Speed Keto

Almost all dairy is restricted

On the Living Speed Keto menu plan we've included up to 2 tsp of heavy cream in a cup of coffee up to a maximum of three times a day; that's it! If you can drink your coffee without cream then so much the better.

We've found that people can be sensitive to dairy, often without knowing it. You don't have to have a full-blown allergy to a particular food to be sensitive to it. However, the irritation it causes when ingested results in inflammation in the body and that inflammation will cause fatigue and slow down weight loss. When weight loss stalls often dairy foods are the culprit. This includes cheese.

I've seen this often enough that I recommend no dairy in my Speed Keto book and I continue this recommendation for those of you who are starting out on this Living Speed Keto program. But don't despair; you can try introducing dairy products after completing a month of Living Speed Keto, paying close attention to how you react.

Testing for dairy intolerance

Follow these instructions to test for dairy intolerance once the first month is over:

- Weigh yourself first thing in the morning
- Eat a small amount of dairy
- Weigh yourself again in the evening

If you see a weight gain (which will be water retention), it's highly likely that dairy products are problematic for you. You can try this test once again after another month of dairy-free eating. If you get the same result then it's best for you to avoid dairy completely.

Nix on excess sweeteners (just for 31 days)

Low-carb sweeteners can also slow down weight loss for some people, so we want you to go easy on sweeteners for the first month of Living Speed Keto. A few of the program recipes do use small amounts of our recommended sweeteners, but this use is limited.

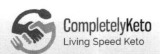

No to alcohol

When alcohol is consumed it is converted by your body into acetate which can then be burned for energy. In fact, your body will switch from burning ketones to using up the acetate in order to get rid of it as soon as possible. Acetate can't be stored so body fat burning stops, ketone production slows down and acetate becomes the prime source of fuel until you stop feeding your body the alcohol.

And here's something else to consider. If you happen to be having a glass of wine with your meal, your liver will be busy making acetate from the alcohol. That will be its priority, so guess what that means? The food you eat will have to be converted to body fat while your liver is otherwise occupied.

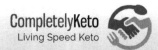

Chapter 3

"YES" Food

Meat

- Bear
- Beef
- Buffalo
- Elk
- Goat
- Lamb
- Pork
- Rabbit
- Venison

Poultry

- Chicken
- Duck
- Goose
- Game hen
- Ostrich
- Partridge
- Pheasant
- Quail
- Squab
- Turkey

Fish

- Ahi
- Catfish
- Cod
- Haddock
- Halibut
- Herring
- Mackerel
- Mahi Mahi
- Salmon
- Sardines
- Snapper
- Swordfish
- Tilapia
- Trout
- Tuna
- Walleye
- White fish

Seafood

- Clams
- Crab
- Lobster
- Mussels
- Oyster
- Prawn
- Scallop
- Scampi
- Shrimp

Fats

On the Living Speed Keto 31-day program, it is important to eat the right (healthy) kind of fats. We burn healthy fats as fuel. Look for and use fats that contain a high amount of saturated fatty acids, also called SFAs. Avoid those high in polyunsaturated fat (PUFA) content whenever you can. The essential fatty-acids contained in PUFAs are important in a healthy diet but it's also important that these "essentials" be eaten in the correct proportions, one-part omega-6 to 4 parts omega-3 (1:4). Most seed and vegetable oils are higher in omega-6 and so we recommend avoiding them.

Our recommended list of fats high in saturated fatty acids and lower in polyunsaturated fats follows:

- MCT oil (97% SFA, less than 1% PUFA) Can be heated - use at low to moderate temperature, no higher than 320 F
- Coconut oil (92% SFA, 1.9% PUFA) Can be heated - use for cooking at higher temperatures
- Cocoa butter (60% SFA, 3% PUFA) Can be heated - use for cooking at higher temperatures
- Beef Tallow (49.8% SFA, 1.3% PUFA) Can be heated - use for cooking at higher temperatures
- Lard (41% SFA, 12% PUFA) Can be heated - use for cooking at higher temperatures
- Duck Fat (25% SFA, 13% PUFA) Can be heated - use for cooking at higher temperatures
- Extra-virgin olive oil (14% SFA, 9.9% PUFA) Use only at low heat temperatures or at room temperature as in salad dressings
- Palm Kernel Oil (82% SFA, 2% PUFA) Can be heated - use for cooking at higher temperatures
- Grass-fed ghee (48% SFA, 4% PUFA) Can be heated - use for cooking at higher temperatures

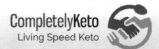

CompletelyKeto
Living Speed Keto

Fruit

In truth, the majority of fruit is very high in natural sugars so their carbohydrate count is too high for them to be included in a ketogenic eating plan. However, there are a few fruits we can include and mostly they are the ones we don't usually think of when considering fruit. Here's a list of the fruits you can include on Living Speed Keto:

- Avocado
- Lemon
- Lime
- Olives
- Tomato (keep this to a minimum)
- Vegetables
- Arugula
- Asparagus
- Bok choy
- Broccoli

- Cabbage
- Capers
- Cauliflower
- Celery
- Collard greens
- Cucumbers
- Eggplant
- Endive
- Garlic
- Kale
- Kelp

- Lettuce
- Mushrooms
- Onions (scallions, red, yellow, white)
- Peppers
- Radishes
- Seaweed
- Spinach
- Swiss chard
- Watercress
- Zucchini

Vegetables to eat in smaller quantities ...

We've included the following vegetables but urge you to use them in smaller amounts as they are higher in carbohydrates than the veggies in the above list.

- Brussels sprouts
- Green beans
- Squash
- Pumpkin

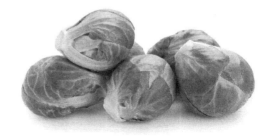

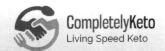

Beverages

Coffee drinking should be kept to a minimum; no more than three cups a day. Caffeine can interfere with weight loss for some people. If you are in a stall, try cutting out caffeine completely (this means coffee and green teas). Make sure to drink plenty of water daily. If you can, drink reverse osmosis water.

- Green tea
- Herbal tea
- Organic coffee
- Organic water processed decaffeinated coffee
- Mineral water
- Water

Natural Sweeteners

We allow two sweeteners on Speed Keto:

- Erythritol (natural sweetener found in some fermented foods and fruits)
- Liquid Stevia (use the liquid stevia not the granular because the granulated stevia may contain maltodextrin which has an extremely high glycemic index)
- Stevia Glycerate (has a thick honey-like texture and tends to not have a bitter after-taste like some other forms of stevia)
- Powdered stevia (very concentrated powder – a little bit goes a long way!)

Erythritol is a sugar alcohol that is found in some fruits and fermented foods. Commercially available erythritol is made from corn. Look for a non-GMO erythritol if you choose to use this sweetener. It's worth noting that not everyone tolerates erythritol well. It can cause diarrhea, headaches and stomach aches, so if you are new to using erythritol use it sparingly until you see how you react.

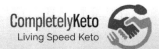

CompletelyKeto
Living Speed Keto

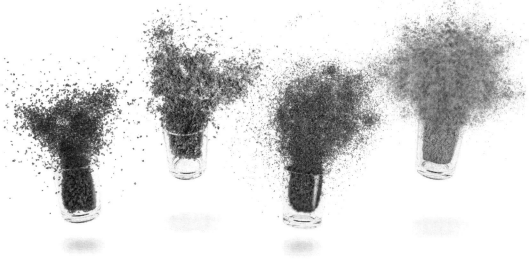

Herbs and Spices

Herbs and spices provide superb nutritional value and add flavor. Use them often!

- Anise
- Basil
- Bay leaf
- Black pepper
- Caraway
- Cardamom
- Cayenne pepper
- Celery seed
- Chervil
- Chili pepper
- Chives
- Cilantro
- Cinnamon
- Cloves
- Coriander
- Cumin
- Curry
- Dill
- Fenugreek
- Galangal
- Garlic
- Ginger
- Lemongrass
- Licorice
- Mace
- Marjoram
- Mint
- Mustard seeds
- Oregano
- Paprika
- Parsley
- Peppermint
- Rosemary
- Saffron
- Sage
- Spearmint
- Star anise
- Tarragon
- Thyme
- Turmeric
- Vanilla beans

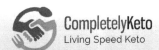

Flavor Enhancers, Sauces and Other Canned Goods

Learn to read labels and then read them all the time. Choose products with no added sugars. It's possible to find things like basic tomato sauce and tomato paste that are made with simple Keto-friendly ingredients, but you have to be vigilant!

- Apple cider vinegar
- White vinegar
- Fish sauce
- Organic tamari
- Boxed organic beef and chicken broth
- Canned anchovies
- Canned coconut milk (full-fat)
- Canned oysters
- Canned sardines
- Canned salmon
- Canned tuna
- Capers
- Fermented pickles (no sugar added)
- Fermented sauerkraut (no sugar added)
- Tomato sauce (no sugar added)
- Tomato paste
- Olives

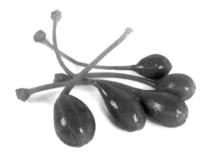

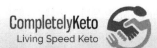

CompletelyKeto
Living Speed Keto

Chapter 4
31 Day Meal Plan

Brief re-cap of how a ketogenic diet works

The Living Speed Keto plan provides delicious ketogenic recipes that will have your body burning fats instead of carbs for energy. The diet you are used to eating is probably heavily reliant on carbohydrates for energy. These carbs are converted into glucose, which is then transported around the body and used as fuel for daily activity including breathing, muscle movements and brain function.

The Living Speed Keto program employs a ketogenic strategy. Because few carbohydrates are included in this meal plan, your liver will quickly switch into converting ingested fat as well as excess body fat into fatty acids and ketones.

Ketones can be easily used by the brain and once the body becomes keto adapted, they quickly replace glucose as the main usable fuel source. It's simply a more efficient way to burn excess body fat and to maintain body weight.

If you are already a client that's been using the Speed Keto program you will enjoy the new recipes my team and I have developed. A few recipes that have been favorites on our website and Facebook page are also included here as well as a few from our specialty collections.

Before you start a quick word about substitutions ...

You will be more successful if you enjoy each mouthful, so substitutions are allowed; with one caveat. You must only substitute using recipes that are provided on the program. If you prefer one meal over another then that's what you should have. If the spice profile of a dish doesn't suit, then change it up for something that does appeal. Swap mixed greens for baby spinach leaves in a salad if that tickles your fancy. The main thing here is to enjoy the meals you eat.

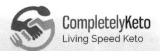
CompletelyKeto
Living Speed Keto

Substitutions will definitely alter the macros (nutritional content) of your meals and may impact your net carb intake for the day, but I wouldn't be too concerned about that. As long as you exchange for allowed food items the substitutions shouldn't be overly significant.

Getting Ready ...

I know you are excited to get started but there are a few things we recommend before diving in:

- Read through the chapters of this book so you understand the principles and science behind the ketogenic lifestyle
- Familiarize yourself with the concept of intermittent fasting and why it works so successfully with a ketogenic meal plan for those wanting to lose weight while gaining energy
- Consult with your doctor
- Make a firm decision to commit to one month of Living Speed Keto

Getting Set ...

There are still a few more items to check off of your to-do list:

It's time to clean out the fridge and pantry. Remove everything on the NO List. The old adage "out of sight, out of mind" applies here!

Purchase any necessary supplements and order online or direct purchase the staple items you need to have on hand for use throughout the month.

Print the calendar style, one-page menu plan and put it somewhere in the kitchen where it will be visible at a glance.

Got everything done? Great!

Now it's time to ...

Get Going!

In order to get going, your first day of Living Speed Keto will also be your preparation day. Every week begins with a prep day that will help you to get set up for the week ahead.

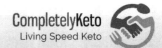
CompletelyKeto
Living Speed Keto

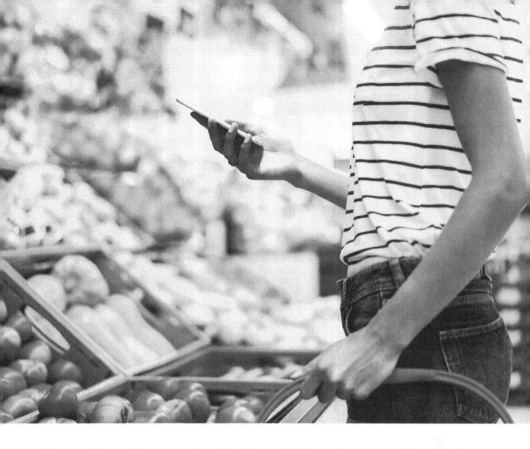

Review the weekly grocery list, check your fridge and pantry and shop for the items you need for this week's recipes.

If you do choose to fast, prepare the homemade chicken broth that will nourish you on these days you (you can also opt to purchase organic broth made from free-range chickens).

If you have a busy schedule you may want to prepare more than one dinner today. Freeze portions that are easy to handle on evenings when you have a lot to do.

Recipes for daily meals are all found at the end of this chapter. An index for each of these recipes have been created for ease of use.

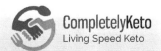

Eating Plan and Menus: Week I

Day #1

This is your first preparation day:

- Weigh yourself, record your weight then put your scales away for the month!
- Measure yourself around the chest, waist, hips, thighs (around both when standing with them together), around one thigh alone and around the upper arm
- Make or buy chicken broth for drinking on intermittent fast days in the week ahead
- Shop for groceries needed to prepare the meals this week
- If necessary, plan for busy days by preparing meals ahead and freezing meal-sized portions

Start your day with Bullet Proof Coffee:

- 1 cup of coffee with 1 tsp MCT oil and, if desired, 2 tsp heavy cream

Menu for the day:

- Breakfast: Keto Eggs Benny
- Lunch: Tuna Salad on Romaine with sliced cucumber & olives
- Dinner: Grilled Flank Steak with Asian Slaw
- Beverages as desired throughout the day: electrolyte drink, water, tea, herbal tea, coffee.

** (no more than 2 tsp of heavy cream per cup in either tea or coffee and no more than 3 cups/day)

Day #2

Start your day with Bullet Proof Coffee:

- 1 cup of coffee with 1 tsp MCT oil and, if desired, 2 tsp heavy cream

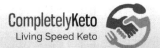

CompletelyKeto
Living Speed Keto

Menu for the day:

- Breakfast: Blueberry Avocado Smoothie
- Lunch: Curried Deviled Eggs
- Dinner: Fiesta Chicken Bowl
- Beverages as desired throughout the day: electrolyte drink, water, tea, herbal tea, coffee.

** (no more than 2 tsp of heavy cream per cup in either tea or coffee and no more than 3 cups/day)

Day #3

Last night you may have begun your first intermittent fast of 42 – 66 hours. If so, today you will be continuing the fast. Start your day by drinking electrolytes followed by a 30-minute walk to deplete glycogen stores.

You may then enjoy a Bulletproof Coffee:

- 1 cup of coffee with 1 tsp MCT Oil and if desired, 2 tsp heavy cream

For the rest of the day, sip on chicken broth as desired. You may also drink the allowed beverages: electrolyte drink (as needed), water, tea, herbal tea and coffee as desired. However, on fasting days drink only clear tea and coffee (no heavy cream). The only cream you can have today is in your morning cup of Bulletproof Coffee.

Menu for the day:

- Breakfast: Fasting (electrolytes, chicken broth, water, coffee, tea)
- Lunch: Fasting (electrolytes, chicken broth, water, coffee, tea)
- Dinner: Fasting (electrolytes, chicken broth, water, coffee, tea)
- Beverages as desired throughout the day: electrolyte drink, water, tea, herbal tea, coffee.

** (no more than 2 tsp of heavy cream per cup in either tea or coffee and no more than 3 cups/day)

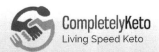

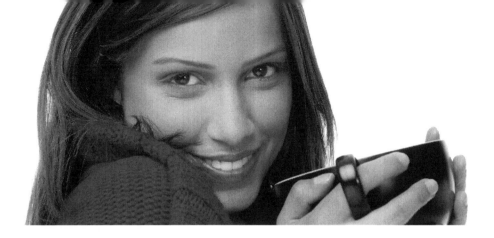

Day #4

This morning you will be continuing the fast.

Start your day with Bullet Proof Coffee:

- 1 cup of coffee with 1 tsp MCT Oil and, if desired, 2 tsp heavy cream

Menu for the day:

- Breakfast: Fasting
- Lunch: Fasting or after 2:00 p.m. - Italian Wedding Soup
- Dinner: Fasting or Pork & Broccoli Stir-fry
- Beverages as desired throughout the day: electrolyte drink, water, tea, herbal tea, coffee.

** (no more than 2 tsp of heavy cream per cup in either tea or coffee and no more than 3 cups/day)

Day #5

If you've chosen to continue fasting until 2:00 pm you will

Start your day by drinking electrolytes followed by a 30-minute walk to deplete glycogen stores. You may then enjoy a Bulletproof Coffee.

- 1 cup of coffee with 1 tsp MCT Oil and, if desired, 2 tsp heavy cream

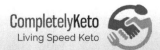

CompletelyKeto
Living Speed Keto

You can also sip on chicken broth as desired and drink the allowed beverages: electrolyte drink (as needed), water, tea, herbal tea and coffee as desired (no heavy cream) until 2 pm.

Everyone else will have the usual Bulletproof Coffee in the morning and three meals today.

- 1 cup of coffee with 1 tsp MCT Oil and, if desired, 2 tsp heavy cream

Menu for the day:

- Breakfast: Fasting or Perfectly Boiled Eggs
- Lunch: Italian Wedding Soup (leftover) or alternate choice from provided Lunch Recipes.
- Dinner: Spaghetti Bolognese
- Beverages as desired throughout the day: electrolyte drink, water, tea, herbal tea, coffee.

** (no more than 2 tsp of heavy cream per cup in either tea or coffee and no more than 3 cups/day)

Day #6

Today you will be having two meals; breakfast and dinner. You may want to have your Bulletproof Coffee in the afternoon as you won't be having lunch today.

Menu for the day:

- Breakfast: Mocha Smoothie
- Lunch: Fasting (have a BPC in the afternoon as well as electrolytes, chicken broth, water, coffee, tea)
- Dinner: Simple Roast Chicken with Steamed Cauliflower & Broccoli
- Beverages as desired throughout the day: electrolyte drink, water, tea, herbal tea, coffee.

** (no more than 2 tsp of heavy cream per cup in either tea or coffee and no more than 3 cups/day)

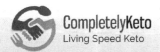

CompletelyKeto
Living Speed Keto

Day #7

Today you may drink Bulletproof Coffee in the morning and enjoy three meals. We also recommend taking a 30-minute walk sometime during the day.

Start your day with Bullet Proof Coffee:

- 1 cup of coffee with 1 tsp MCT Oil and, if desired, 2 tsp heavy cream

Menu for the day:

- Breakfast: Keto Pancakes with Lakanto syrup
- Lunch: Spinach Salad with Chicken (chicken left-over from last night's dinner)
- Dinner: Roasted Turkey Breast with Cauliflower Mash plus salad & dressing of choice
- Beverages as desired throughout the day: electrolyte drink, water, tea, herbal tea, coffee.

** *(no more than 2 tsp of heavy cream per cup in either tea or coffee and no more than 3 cups/day)*

Week II

Day #8

It's prep day again.

Today you will be eating three meals but tomorrow OMAD begins. For the next 4 days you will be eating one meal a day. This is a form of intermittent fasting with a 23 hour fasting period between meals. So, there will be way less prep for the week to come. However, there is a bit to accomplish before bedtime rolls around today.

We suggest you make another big pot of chicken broth. You can have a cup as needed throughout the day on OMAD. Keep 3 days worth in the fridge and freeze the remainder in single sized portion containers for easy use.

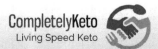

CompletelyKeto
Living Speed Keto

You will also need to review the recipes for this week and restock the fridge and pantry with needed items. If it's a busy week coming up you could also pre-prepare meals and freeze them in appropriately portioned sizes. But today you will enjoy three meals before OMAD begins.

Start your day with Bullet Proof Coffee:

- 1 cup of coffee with 1 tsp MCT Oil and, if desired, 2 tsp heavy cream

Menu for the day:

- Breakfast: Poached Egg with Hollandaise on Asparagus
- Lunch: Turkey Buddha Lunch Bowl with Vinaigrette
- Dinner: Baked Whole Fish with Baby Bok Choy Stir-fry
- Beverages as desired throughout the day: electrolyte drink, water, tea, herbal tea, coffee.

*** (no more than 2 tsp of heavy cream per cup in either tea or coffee and no more than 3 cups/day)*

Day #9

It's an OMAD day so you will be having a satisfying dinner this evening.

Start your day with Bullet Proof Coffee:

- 1 cup of coffee with 1 tsp MCT Oil and, if desired, 2 tsp heavy cream

Menu for the day:

- Breakfast: Fasting (electrolytes, chicken broth, water, coffee, tea)
- Lunch: Fasting (electrolytes, chicken broth, water, coffee, tea)
- Dinner: Keto Chili with salad & dressing of your choice
- Beverages as desired throughout the day: electrolyte drink, water, tea, herbal tea, coffee.

*** (no more than 2 tsp of heavy cream per cup in either tea or coffee and no more than 3 cups/day)*

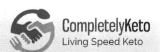

CompletelyKeto
Living Speed Keto

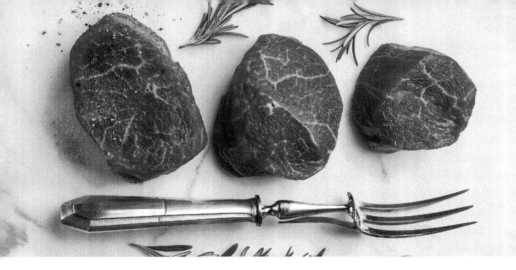

Day #10

It's an OMAD day so you will be having a satisfying dinner this evening.

Start your day with Bullet Proof Coffee:

- 1 cup of coffee with 1 tsp MCT Oil and, if desired, 2 tsp heavy cream.

Menu for the day:

- Breakfast: fasting (BPC, electrolytes, chicken broth, water, coffee, tea)
- Lunch: fasting (BPC, electrolytes, chicken broth, water, coffee, tea)
- Dinner: Perfect Steak with Plattered Tomato Salad
- Beverages as desired throughout the day: electrolyte drink, water, tea, herbal tea, coffee.

*** (no more than 2 tsp of heavy cream per cup in either tea or coffee and no more than 3 cups/day)*

Day #11

OMAD today, so you will be having a satisfying dinner this evening.

Start your day with Bullet Proof Coffee:

- 1 cup of coffee with 1 tsp MCT Oil and, if desired, 2 tsp heavy cream

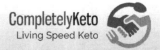
CompletelyKeto
Living Speed Keto

Menu for the day:

- Breakfast: Fasting (electrolytes, chicken broth, water, coffee, tea)
- Lunch: Fasting- (electrolytes, chicken broth, water, coffee, tea)
- Dinner: Harlan's Red Thai Curry Chicken Soup
- Beverages as desired throughout the day: electrolyte drink, water, tea, herbal tea, coffee.

*** (no more than 2 tsp of heavy cream per cup in either tea or coffee and no more than 3 cups/day)*

Day #12

OMAD today, so you will be having a satisfying dinner this evening.

Start your day with Bullet Proof Coffee:

- 1 cup of coffee with 1 tsp MCT Oil and, if desired, 2 tsp heavy cream

Menu for the day:

- Breakfast: Fasting (electrolytes, chicken broth, water, coffee, tea)
- Lunch: Fasting (electrolytes, chicken broth, water, coffee, tea)
- Dinner: Harlan's Chicken Saltimbocca with Roasted Brussels Sprouts
- Beverages as desired throughout the day: electrolyte drink, water, tea, herbal tea, coffee.

*** (no more than 2 tsp of heavy cream per cup in either tea or coffee and no more than 3 cups/day)*

Day #13

Two meals today; breakfast and dinner.

Start your day as usual with Bullet Proof Coffee:

- 1 cup of coffee with 1 tsp MCT Oil and, if desired, 2 tsp heavy cream

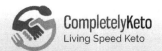

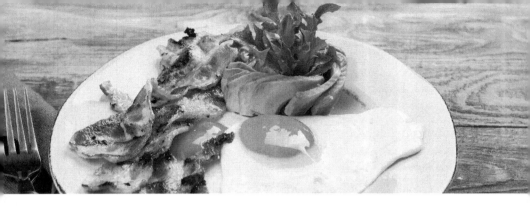

Menu for the day:

- Breakfast: Bacon & Eggs with avocado
- Lunch: Fasting (Electrolytes, chicken broth, water, coffee, tea)
- Dinner: Seared Scallops with Sautéed Asparagus
- Beverages as desired throughout the day: electrolyte drink, water, tea, herbal tea, coffee.

** (no more than 2 tsp of heavy cream per cup in either tea or coffee and no more than 3 cups/day)

Day #14

Three meals today!

Start your day with Bullet Proof Coffee:

- 1 cup of coffee with 1 tsp MCT Oil and, if desired, 2 tsp heavy cream

Menu for the day:

- Breakfast: Baked Eggs Florentine
- Lunch: Old Fashioned Chicken Noodle Soup
- Dinner: Lamb Souvlaki with Harlan's Israeli Salad
- Beverages as desired throughout the day: electrolyte drink, water, tea, herbal tea, coffee.

** (no more than 2 tsp of heavy cream per cup in either tea or coffee and no more than 3 cups/day)

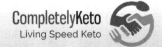

CompletelyKeto
Living Speed Keto

Week III

Day #15

It's prep day again. Today you will need to get ready for the week ahead:

- Make or buy chicken broth for drinking on intermittent fasting days
- Shop for groceries needed to prepare the meals this week
- If necessary, plan for busy days by preparing meals ahead and freezing meal-sized portions.

Start your day with Bullet Proof Coffee:

- 1 cup of coffee with 1 tsp MCT Oil and, if desired, 2 tsp heavy cream

Menu for the day:

- Breakfast: Keto Pancakes with Lakanto Syrup
- Lunch: Old Fashioned Chicken Noodle Soup (left-over)
- Dinner: Crispy Skin Salmon Fillet with salad & dressing of your choice
- Beverages as desired throughout the day: electrolyte drink, water, tea, herbal tea, coffee.

*** (no more than 2 tsp of heavy cream per cup in either tea or coffee and no more than 3 cups/day)*

Day #16

Today you may drink Bulletproof Coffee in the morning and enjoy three meals. No eating past 8:00 pm (first period of intermittent fasting begins) however hydration with water is allowed.

Start your day with Bullet Proof Coffee:

- 1 cup of coffee with 1 tsp MCT Oil and, if desired, 2 tsp heavy cream

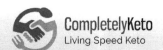

CompletelyKeto
Living Speed Keto

Menu for the day:

- Breakfast: Mocha Smoothie
- Lunch: Tuna Salad on Romaine with sliced cucumber & olives
- Dinner: Baked Baby Back Ribs with Mock Potato Salad
- No eating or snacks after 8 p.m. (fast of 42-66 hours begins)
- Beverages as desired throughout the day: electrolyte drink, water, tea, herbal tea, coffee.

*** (no more than 2 tsp of heavy cream per cup in either tea or coffee and no more than 3 cups/day)*

Day #17

Last night you began an intermittent fast of 42-66 hours. Today you will be continuing the fast.

Start your day with Bullet Proof Coffee:

- 1 cup of coffee with 1 tsp MCT Oil and, if desired, 2 tsp heavy cream

Menu for the day:

- Breakfast: Fasting
- Lunch: Fasting
- Dinner: Fasting
- Beverages as desired throughout the day: electrolyte drink, water, tea, herbal tea, coffee.

*** (no more than 2 tsp of heavy cream per cup in either tea or coffee and no more than 3 cups/day)*

Day #18

This morning you will be continuing the fast. Start your day by drinking electrolytes followed by:

- 30-minute walk to deplete glycogen stores

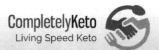

CompletelyKeto
Living Speed Keto

You may then enjoy a Bulletproof Coffee:

- 1 cup of coffee with 1 tsp MCT Oil and, if desired, 2 tsp heavy cream

Today you will have a decision to make. You may eat lunch after 2:00 pm (42 hour fast) or continue fasting until tomorrow at 2:00 pm (66 hour fast). If you choose to continue fasting until tomorrow you will sip on chicken broth as desired and drink the allowed beverages: electrolyte drink (as needed), water, tea, herbal tea and coffee as desired (no heavy cream).

If you choose to end your fasting period at 2:00 pm you will be eating two meals today; lunch and dinner.

Start your day with Bullet Proof Coffee:

- 1 cup of coffee with 1 tsp MCT Oil and, if desired, 2 tsp heavy cream

Menu for the day:

- Breakfast: Fasting
- Lunch: Fasting - may decide to continue through tomorrow OR until 2:00 pm, then Italian Wedding Soup
- Dinner: Fasting – may decide to continue through tomorrow OR, Tex/Mex Fish Roll-ups with Everyday Green Salad
- Beverages as desired throughout the day: electrolyte drink, water, tea, herbal tea, coffee.

Day #19

If you've chosen to continue fasting until 2:00 pm you will: Start your day by drinking electrolytes followed by ...

- a 30-minute walk to deplete glycogen stores

You may then enjoy a Bulletproof Coffee:

- 1 cup of coffee with 1 tsp MCT Oil and, if desired, 2 tsp heavy cream

You can also sip on chicken broth as desired and drink the allowed beverages: electrolyte drink, water, tea, herbal tea and coffee as desired (no heavy cream) until 2 pm.

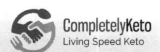

CompletelyKeto
Living Speed Keto

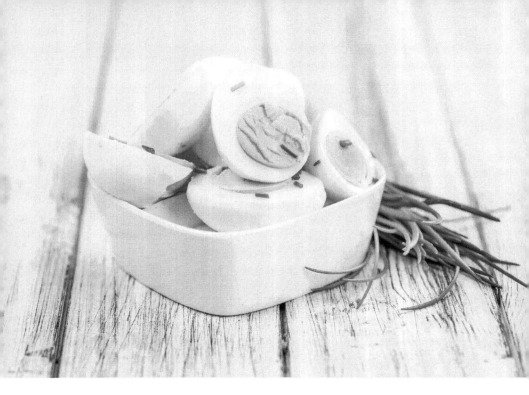

Everyone else will have the usual Bulletproof Coffee in the morning and three meals today.

Menu for the day:

- Breakfast: Fasting or Chana's Speed Keto Thick Milk Shake
- Lunch: Left-over Italian Wedding Soup (or choose an alternate lunch from our Lunch Recipes)
- Dinner: Spatchcocked Chicken & Cauliflower Mash with Garlic and Plattered Tomato Salad
- Beverages as desired throughout the day: electrolyte drink, water, tea, herbal tea, coffee.

*** (no more than 2 tsp of heavy cream per cup in either tea or coffee and no more than 3 cups/day)*

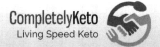

Day #20

Today you will be having two meals; breakfast and dinner. You may want to have your Bulletproof Coffee in the afternoon as you won't be having lunch today.

Start your day with Bullet Proof Coffee:

- 1 cup of coffee with 1 tsp MCT Oil and, if desired, 2 tsp heavy cream

Menu for the day:

- Breakfast: Perfectly Boiled Eggs
- Lunch: Fasting (have a BPC in the afternoon)
- Dinner: Fiesta Chicken Bowl (use leftover chicken from last night)
- Beverages as desired throughout the day: electrolyte drink, water, tea, herbal tea, coffee.

*** (no more than 2 tsp of heavy cream per cup in either tea or coffee and no more than 3 cups/day)*

Day #21

Today you will be having two meals; breakfast and dinner. You may want to have your Bulletproof Coffee in the afternoon as you won't be having lunch today.

Start your day with Bullet Proof Coffee:

- 1 cup of coffee with 1 tsp MCT Oil and, if desired, 2 tsp heavy cream

Menu for the day:

- Breakfast: Mocha Smoothie
- Lunch: Curried Deviled Eggs with sliced tomato and/or cucumber
- Dinner: Grilled Flank Steak with Caesar Salad for Two
- Beverages as desired throughout the day: electrolyte drink, water, tea, herbal tea, coffee.

*** (no more than 2 tsp of heavy cream per cup in either tea or coffee and no more than 3 cups/day)*

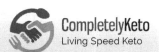

CompletelyKeto
Living Speed Keto

Week IV

Day #22

It's prep day again. Today you will be eating three meals but tomorrow OMAD begins. For the next 4 days you will be eating one meal a day. This is a form of intermittent fasting with a 24-hour fasting period between meals. So, there will be way less prep for the week to come. However, there is a bit to accomplish before bedtime rolls around today: We suggest you make another big pot of chicken broth. You can have a cup as needed throughout the day on OMAD. Keep 3 days worth in the fridge and freeze the remainder in single sized portion containers for easy use. You will also need to review the recipes for this week and restock the fridge and pantry with needed items. If it's a busy week coming up you could also pre-prepare meals and freeze them in appropriately portioned sizes. Also try to get out and have a 20 minute walk at some point. Enjoy three meals today.

Start your day with Bullet Proof Coffee:

- 1 cup of coffee with 1 tsp MCT Oil and, if desired, 2 tsp heavy cream

Menu for the day:

- Breakfast: Baked Eggs Florentine
- Lunch: Spinach Salad with Chicken
- Dinner: Fish Fry with Turnip "Fries" & Keto Slaw
- Beverages as desired throughout the day: electrolyte drink, water, tea, herbal tea, coffee.

** *(no more than 2 tsp of heavy cream per cup in either tea or coffee and no more than 3 cups/day)*

Day #23

It's an OMAD day so you will be having a satisfying dinner this evening. Start your day with Bullet Proof Coffee:

- 1 cup of coffee with 1 tsp MCT Oil and, if desired, 2 tsp heavy cream

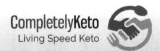

CompletelyKeto
Living Speed Keto

Menu for the day:

- Breakfast: Fasting (electrolytes, chicken broth, water, coffee and tea throughout the day)
- Lunch: Fasting (electrolytes, chicken broth, water, coffee and tea throughout the day)
- Dinner: Keto Chili with Every Day Green Salad
- Beverages as desired throughout the day: electrolyte drink, water, tea, herbal tea, coffee.

** (no more than 2 tsp of heavy cream per cup in either tea or coffee and no more than 3 cups/day)

Day #24

It's an OMAD day so you will be having a satisfying dinner this evening. Start your day with Bullet Proof Coffee:

- 1 cup of coffee with 1 tsp MCT Oil and, if desired, 2 tsp heavy cream

Menu for the day:

- Breakfast: Fasting (electrolytes, chicken broth, water, coffee and tea throughout the day)
- Lunch: Fasting (electrolytes, chicken broth, water, coffee and tea throughout the day)
- Dinner: Harlan's Thai Red Curry Chicken Soup
- Beverages as desired throughout the day: electrolyte drink, water, tea, herbal tea, coffee.

** (no more than 2 tsp of heavy cream per cup in either tea or coffee and no more than 3 cups/day)

Day #25

It's an OMAD day so you will be having a satisfying dinner this evening. Start your day with Bullet Proof Coffee:

- 1 cup of coffee with 1 tsp MCT Oil and, if desired, 2 tsp heavy cream

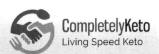

Menu for the day:
- Breakfast: Fasting (electrolytes, chicken broth, water, coffee and tea throughout the day)
- Lunch: Fasting (electrolytes, chicken broth, water, coffee and tea throughout the day)
- Dinner: Lamb Souvlaki with Harlan's Israeli Salad
- Beverages as desired throughout the day: electrolyte drink, water, tea, herbal tea, coffee.

*** (no more than 2 tsp of heavy cream per cup in either tea or coffee and no more than 3 cups/day)*

Day #26

It's an OMAD day so you will be having a satisfying dinner this evening. Start your day with Bullet Proof Coffee:

- 1 cup of coffee with 1 tsp MCT Oil and, if desired, 2 tsp heavy cream.

Menu for the day:
- Breakfast: Fasting (electrolytes, chicken broth, water, coffee and tea throughout the day)
- Lunch: Fasting (electrolytes, chicken broth, water, coffee and tea throughout the day)
- Dinner: Spaghetti Bolognese
- Beverages as desired throughout the day: electrolyte drink, water, tea, herbal tea, coffee.

*** (no more than 2 tsp of heavy cream per cup in either tea or coffee and no more than 3 cups/day)*

Day #27

Today you will be having two meals.

Start your day with Bullet Proof Coffee:

- 1 cup of coffee with 1 tsp MCT Oil and, if desired, 2 tsp heavy cream

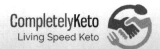
CompletelyKeto
Living Speed Keto

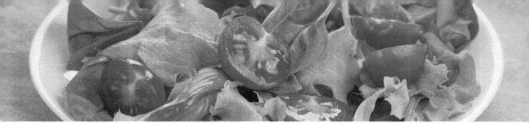

Menu for the day:

- Breakfast: Baked Eggs in Avocado with Smoked Salmon
- Lunch: Fasting - electrolytes, chicken broth, water, coffee and tea throughout the day
- Dinner: Roasted Turkey Breast with Cauliflower "Rice" and salad of choice
- Beverages as desired throughout the day: electrolyte drink, water, tea, herbal tea, coffee.

** (no more than 2 tsp of heavy cream per cup in either tea or coffee and no more than 3 cups/day)

Day #28

Today you may drink Bulletproof Coffee in the morning and enjoy three meals. We also recommend taking a 30-minute walk sometime during the day.

Start your day with Bullet Proof Coffee:

- 1 cup of coffee with 1 tsp MCT Oil and, if desired, 2 tsp heavy cream

Menu for the day:

- Breakfast: Mocha Smoothie
- Lunch: Turkey Buddha Lunch Bowl (use left-over turkey from last night) with Vinaigrette
- Dinner: Pork & Broccoli Stir-fry
- Beverages as desired throughout the day: electrolyte drink, water, tea, herbal tea, coffee.

** (no more than 2 tsp of heavy cream per cup in either tea or coffee and no more than 3 cups/day)

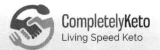

Week V

Day #29

You are almost there ... just three more days and you will have completed the month-long Speed Keto program. Today you will have three meals. Complete your eating for the day and be ready to begin fasting by 8:00 pm this evening. You will fast tomorrow and the next day until 2:00 pm.

Today is prep day:

We suggest you make another big pot of chicken broth. You can have a cup Keep 3 days worth in the fridge and freeze the remainder in single sized portion containers for easy use. You will also need to review the recipes for this week and restock the fridge and pantry with needed items. If it's a busy week coming up you could also pre-prepare meals and freeze them in appropriately portioned sizes. Also try to get out and have a 30-minute walk at some point. Enjoy three meals today

Start your day with Bullet Proof Coffee:

- 1 cup of coffee with 1 tsp MCT Oil and, if desired, 2 tsp heavy cream

Menu for the day:

- Breakfast: Keto Pancakes & Lakanto Syrup
- Lunch: Poached Egg with Hollandaise on Asparagus
- Dinner: Simple Roast Chicken with Cauliflower Mash and Roasted Brussels Sprouts
- Beverages as desired throughout the day: electrolyte drink, water, tea, herbal tea, coffee.

** *(no more than 2 tsp of heavy cream per cup in either tea or coffee and no more than 3 cups/day)*

Day #30

Start your day with Bullet Proof Coffee:

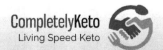

CompletelyKeto
Living Speed Keto

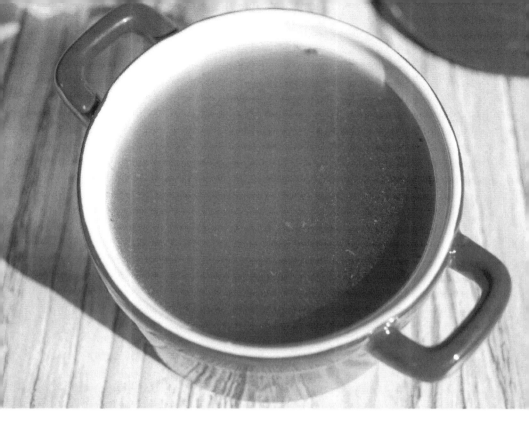

- 1 cup of coffee with 1 tsp MCT Oil and, if desired, 2 tsp heavy cream

Menu for the day:

- Breakfast: Fasting - electrolytes, chicken broth, water, tea throughout the day
- Lunch: Fasting
- Dinner: Fasting
- Beverages as desired throughout the day: electrolyte drink, water, tea, herbal tea, coffee.

** (no more than 2 tsp of heavy cream per cup in either tea or coffee and no more than 3 cups/day)

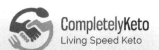

CompletelyKeto
Living Speed Keto

Day #31

Congratulations ... you've made it to the last day of the Living Speed Keto 31-day program. Today you can measure your success! It's time to get out the scales and measuring tape: Weigh yourself Measure yourself around the chest, waist, hips, thigh (around both when standing with them together), around one thigh alone and around the upper arm. Compare to measurements and weight on Day 1. Today you will fast until 2:00 pm.

Start your day with Bullet Proof Coffee:

- 1 cup of coffee with 1 tsp MCT Oil and, if desired, 2 tsp heavy cream

Menu for the day:

- Breakfast: Fasting - electrolytes, chicken broth, water, tea throughout the day
- Lunch: Fast until 2:00 pm then Old Fashioned Chicken Noodle Soup
- Dinner: Crispy Skin Salmon Fillet with Caesar Salad for Two
- Beverages as desired throughout the day: electrolyte drink, water, tea, herbal tea, coffee.

** (no more than 2 tsp of heavy cream per cup in either tea or coffee and no more than 3 cups/day)

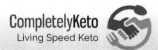

CompletelyKeto
Living Speed Keto

Shopping Lists

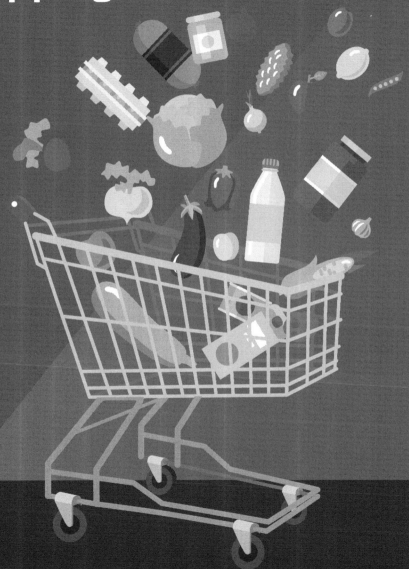

Shopping Lists

I know that shopping for organic fruit & veggies as well as pastured grain fed meats & dairy can be an added expense. Remember there may be somewhere else, other than your weekly food budget, where spending can be trimmed down. Just do your best on this front.

I don't always include amounts with the items on the food lists as some of you may be feeding several people while others are just cooking for one. Have a look at the recipes for each week before you go shopping and alter what you purchase accordingly.

Week I

Basics

- MCT oil
- Coffee (regular & decaffeinated)
- Tea (regular, decaffeinated & herbal)
- Calcium/ magnesium powder (if making homemade electrolyte drink)
- Pink Himalayan salt
- Black pepper corns
- Stevia (concentrated powder form or liquid stevia)
- Erythritol (if using as a sweetener)
- Powdered mustard
- Onion powder
- Curry powder
- Taco seasoning powder
- Dried oregano
- Dried basil
- Dried thyme leaves
- Dried sage
- Smoked paprika
- Bay leaves
- Pure vanilla extract
- Cocoa powder
- Extra-virgin olive oil
- Dark sesame oil
- Ghee (if not making your own)
- Coconut oil
- White vinegar
- Apple cider vinegar

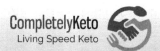

CompletelyKeto
Living Speed Keto

Meat & Poultry

- 1 ½ lb Flank steak
- 2 chickens (only buy one if not making homemade broth)
- Italian sausages
- Ground beef
- 4 leg/thigh chicken quarters (for soup)
- 1 chicken breast (if needed for the chicken Fiesta Bowl)
- Small pork tenderloin
- Bacon (pork or turkey)
- 2 ½ lb turkey breast, skin on

Fruit

- 3 lemons
- 1 lime
- 3 avocado
- Blueberries (fresh or frozen)
- Cherry tomatoes
- Veggies
- 2 bags (or boxes) baby spinach leaves
- 2 Garlic bulbs
- Red onion
- Bag of yellow cooking onions
- 1 package shallots
- 2 small bok choy
- ½ lb cremini mushrooms
- English cucumber
- Celery
- Romaine lettuce (small head)
- 1 head cauliflower
- 1 bunch broccoli
- 1 jalapeño pepper
- 1 red bell pepper
- 2 small zucchini
- 1 bunch flat leaf parsley

Dairy Section

- Heavy cream (if using in coffee)
- 2 doz. large sized eggs

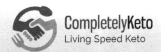

CompletelyKeto
Living Speed Keto

Other

- 2 cans full fat coconut milk
- Canned tuna
- Mediterranean style black olives
- Full-fat mayonnaise
- Dijon mustard

- Lakanto syrup
- Sugar-free hot sauce of choice (sugar-free sriracha, etc.)
- Chicken bouillon cubes &/or boxed chicken broth (if needed)

- 2 packages Miracle Noodle (also known as yam noodle or konjac noodle)
- 8 oz canned tomato sauce (sugar-free)

Week II

Basics

- Chili powder
- Smoked chipotle powder
- Ground cumin

- Poultry seasoning
- Red Thai curry paste
- Nutritional yeast

- White wine vinegar

Meat & Poultry

- 1 Whole chicken, (for making broth if needed)
- 2 boneless, skinless chicken breasts (if need for making Harlan's Thai Red Curry Chicken Soup)
- 2 lb. boneless, skinless chicken

breasts, for Chicken Saltimbocca Recipe
- 4 - leg/thigh chicken quarters (for old Fashioned Chicken Soup recipe)
- 1 lb ground beef or turkey

- 4 filet mignon steaks (or other steaks of your choice)
- 1 ½ lb boneless lamb shoulder
- ¼ lb navel pastrami thinly sliced

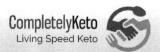

CompletelyKeto
Living Speed Keto

Fish & Seafood

- 4 whole fish – sea bass, trout or bream
- 1 ½ lb large scallops

Dairy Section

- 1 - 2 doz eggs
- Heavy cream (if using in coffee)

Fruit

- 4 lemons
- 1 lime
- Avocado
- Cherry tomatoes
- 4 plum tomatoes
- 2 large tomatoes

Veggies

- 2 lb asparagus spears
- Mixed salad greens
- 1 bag or box baby spinach leaves
- 1 zucchini
- 1 lb Brussels sprouts
- 2 Red bell pepper
- Red chili pepper, select pepper with the level of heat you preference
- 2 jalapeño peppers
- English cucumber
- Lemon grass stalks (or use a lemon cut into slices if you can't get lemon grass)
- 1 bunch fresh basil
- 1 bunch fresh mint
- 1 bunch fresh cilantro
- 12 sage leaves
- Small fresh ginger root
- 4 or 5 small baby bok choy (enough for 4 C chopped)
- 1 or 2 garlic bulb
- Red onion, if needed
- 1 large or 2 small heads cauliflower
- 1 medium tomato
- Small cabbage (or bag of pre-shredded cabbage)
- Celery (if needed)

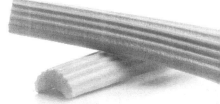

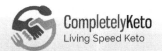

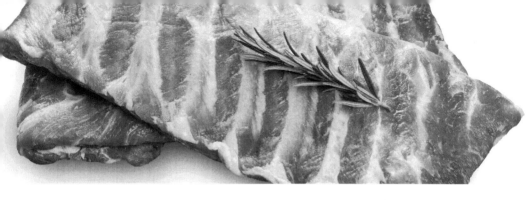

Other

- 1 box organic beef broth
- 2 boxes organic chicken broth
- 1 can tomato paste
- 1 bottle of capers
- 1 can full fat coconut milk
- 1 package "Miracle" noodles
- Pinot Grigio
- Wooden skewers (if needed for lamb souvlaki)

Week III

Basics

- Liquid smoke
- Cinnamon
- Tahini
- Ghee (if needed)
- Anchovy paste (if wanted for Caesar salad)
- Worcestershire sauce (sugar-free)

Meat & Poultry

- 2 full racks baby back ribs
- Italian sausages, large
- 1 or 2 whole chickens (buy 1 if not making homemade)
- 1 ½ lb flank steak

Fish & Seafood

- Salmon (4 fillets, skin on)
- ½ lb firm fleshed white fish (cod, halibut, flounder, haddock)

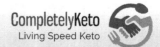

CompletelyKeto
Living Speed Keto

Dairy Section

- Heavy cream (if using in coffee)
- Eggs

Fruit

- 3 lemons
- 1 lime
- 3 avocado

- English cucumber
- 3 medium tomatoes

- Cherry tomatoes

Veggies

- 1 head romaine lettuce
- Arugula
- 2 heads Boston lettuce (or other leaf lettuce), you need 8 large leaves

- 1or 2 bags or boxes of baby spinach leaves
- 1 bag yellow cooking onions (if needed)
- 1 red onion

- 2 bulbs garlic
- 1 bunch scallions (green onions)
- 3 medium heads cauliflower

Other

- Can of solid tuna
- Olives (if needed)
- Can of full fat coconut cream

- 1 box organic chicken stock (for Italian Wedding Soup, if needed)

- 8 oz marinara sauce (sugar-free)

Week IV

Meat & Poultry

- Whole chicken (if making broth)
- 4 boneless, skinless chicken breasts

- Bacon (turkey or pork)
- 2 lbs ground beef or turkey
- 1 ½ lb boneless

- lamb shoulder
- Small pork tenderloin
- 2 ½ lb turkey breast with skin

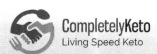

Fish & Seafood

- 2 lb haddock
- 3 oz smoked salmon

Dairy Section

- Eggs
- Heavy cream
- Fruit
- 1 lime
- 4 lemons
- Tomato
- Cherry tomatoes
- 3 avocados
- Veggies
- Large bag or box of Baby spinach leaves

- Mixed greens
- English cucumber
- 4 small turnip
- 1 cabbage or (3 C pre-shredded package)
- Red bell pepper
- Red onion (if needed)
- 2 jalapeño peppers
- 3 Cauliflower
- 1 bunch broccoli

- 1 bunch fresh cilantro
- 1 bunch flat leaf parsley
- 1 bunch fresh mint
- 1 bunch scallions (green onions)
- 2 bulbs garlic
- Ginger root
- Cremini mushrooms
- 3 zucchini

Other

- 2 cans of full fat coconut milk
- Dill Pickles (sugar-free)
- Tomato paste

- 1 can unsweetened tomato sauce
- 1 box organic beef broth

- 6 C organic chicken broth
- 1 package "Miracle" noodles

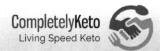

CompletelyKeto
Living Speed Keto

Week V

Meat & Poultry

- 1 or 2 whole chickens (one if not making broth)
- 4 – chicken leg/thigh quarters

Fish & Seafood

- 4 oz salmon fillets, skin on

Dairy Section

- Coffee cream (if needed)
- Eggs (if needed)

Veggies

- 24 asparagus spears
- 1 romaine lettuce
- Arugula
- 1 head cauliflower
- 1 package pre-shredded cabbage or 1 small head
- Celery
- Garlic bulb (if needed)
- Brussels sprouts

Other

- 1 box organic chicken broth
- 1 package "miracle" noodles

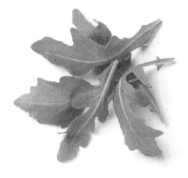

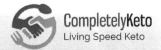

Recipes

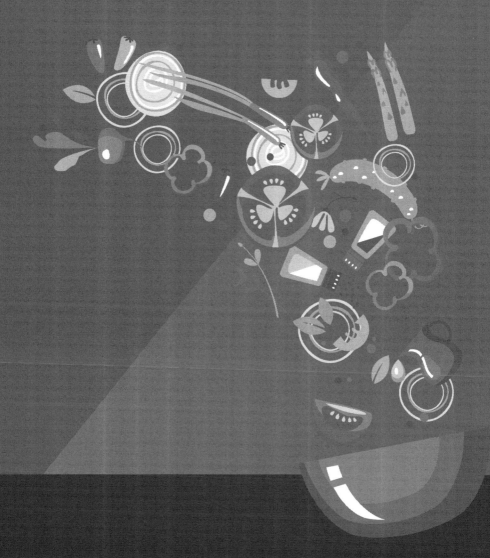

Essentials
Bullet Proof Coffee (BPC)
Homemade Electrolyte Drink
Homemade Chicken Broth
Ghee
Smokey BBQ Sauce

Breakfast
Perfectly Poached Eggs
Keto Eggs Benny
Blueberry Avocado Smoothie
Perfectly Boiled Eggs
Mocha Smoothie
Keto Bread/Bun/ Pancakes!
Poached Egg with Hollandaise on Asparagus
Bacon & Eggs
Baked Eggs Florentine
Chana Kilstein's Speed Keto Thick Shake
Baked Eggs in Avocado with Smoked Salmon

Lunch
Tuna Salad on Romaine (with Sliced Cucumber & Olives)
Curried Deviled Eggs
Italian Wedding Soup
Spinach Salad with Chicken
Turkey Buddha Lunch Bowl
Old fashioned Chicken Noodle Soup

Dinner
Grilled Flank Steak with Asian Slaw
Fiesta Chicken Bowl
Stir-fried Pork & Broccoli
Spaghetti Bolognese
Simple Roast Chicken
Baked Whole Fish; Thai Style
Roasted Turkey Breast
Keto Chili
Perfect Steak
Harlan's Thai Red Curry, Chicken Soup
Harlan's Chicken Saltimbocca
Lamb Souvlaki
Seared Scallops on Sautéed Asparagus
Crispy Skin Salmon Fillet
Oven Baked Baby Back Ribs
Tex/Mex Fish Roll-ups
Roasted Spatchcocked Chicken
Speedy Fish Fry

Veggies & Sides
Zucchini "Noodles"
Steamed Cauliflower & Broccoli
Baby Bok Choy Stir-fry
Cauliflower Mash
Cauliflower Hash Browns
Cauliflower "Rice"
Roasted Brussels Sprouts
Turnip "Fries"

Salads & Dressings
Vinaigrette
Completely Keto Green Goddess Dressing
Keto Coleslaw
Every Day Green Salad
Simple Caesar Salad for Two
Plattered Tomato Salad
Harlan's Israeli Salad
Mock Potato Salad

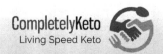

CompletelyKeto
Living Speed Keto

Essential Recipes

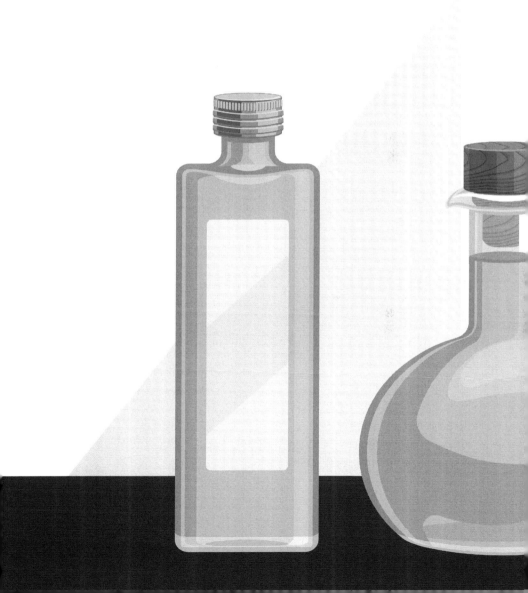

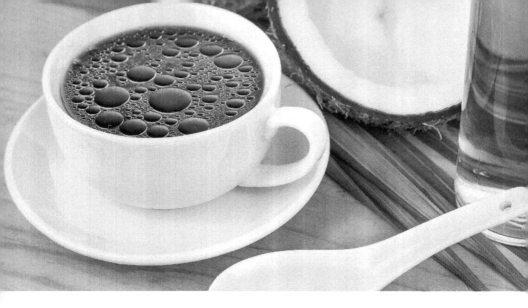

Bullet Proof Coffee

There are many different versions of bullet proof coffee out there on the internet. The Speed Keto version is simple:

- 1 cup of coffee with 1 tsp MCT oil and, if desired, 2 tsp heavy cream.

That's it!

The usual time of day to drink this coffee is first thing in the morning because it immediately introduces an energy source for your body in the form of ketones. It's just a great way to start the day.

Note: Some people react with loose stools when first adding MCT oil to their diet. You will most likely be okay with just one teaspoon but if you notice a problem cut back to ½ tsp and slowly build up to 1 teaspoon in your bullet proof morning coffee.

Nutritional Information:

- Calories/serving: 77 (with cream) ... 45 (without cream)
- Total Carbs: 0
- Fiber: 0
- Total Fats: 8 g (with cream) ... 5 g (without cream)
- Protein: 0

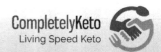

CompletelyKeto
Living Speed Keto

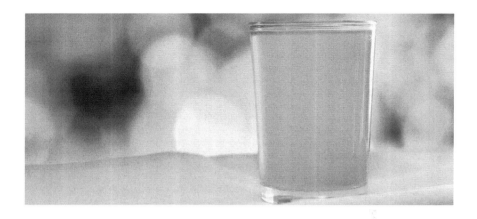

Homemade Electrolyte Drink

There are many brands of electrolyte drinks commercially available today but homemade is also a convenient and more economical option. You can pick up powdered calcium magnesium mixtures at most pharmacies, health food/supplement stores or you can also easily order it from online sources.

I use a fruit flavored herbal tea as a base for my homemade electrolyte brew and steep it with an added stevia leaf for sweetener. I know fresh stevia leaves aren't available to everyone so this recipe includes the option of sweetening to taste with the powdered version.

Ingredients

- 1 quart base liquid (green tea, flavored herbal tea, coconut water, or plain water
- 1/8 -1/4 tsp Himalayan salt
- 1 tsp calcium/magnesium powder
- Stevia sweetener (to taste)

Preparation

1. Brew tea if using, or slightly warm the base liquid.

2. Add Himalayan salt, calcium magnesium and stevia powder (if using). Mix well until the additions have dissolved into the base liquid.

3. Cool and store in refrigerator for up to four days.

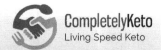
CompletelyKeto
Living Speed Keto

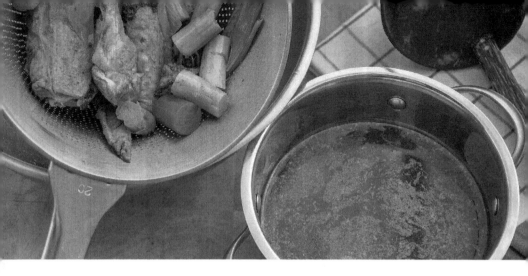

Homemade Chicken Broth

You will want to get the soup pot out in the morning because this chicken stock will spend 5-6 hours on your stove-top before it's really done. The long slow simmer maximizes the nutritional value and deepens flavor. Some of the broth will be consumed during fasting this week so you will be appreciating these amazing flavors soon!

When the internal temperature of the chicken reaches 185 F the meat is cooked. The chicken meat can be used for dinner with the bones from the carcass going back into the pot for the rest of the simmer time, 5-8 hours (or more). Makes about 4 quarts of stock.

Ingredients

- 1, 4-5 lb chicken whole or cut into pieces
- 2 celery stalks cut in half
- 5 garlic cloves, smashed open or cut in half
- 1 large bay leaf
- 3-5 sprigs fresh thyme (or 1 ½ tsp dried)
- Handful of fresh parsley (or 2 tsp dried)
- 2 tsp sea salt
- 1 tsp black peppercorns
- 1 ½ T apple cider vinegar
- Water to fill the 6-8 quart pot

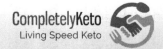

CompletelyKeto
Living Speed Keto

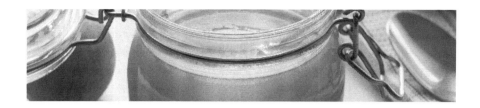

Homemade Chicken Broth (continued)

Preparation

1. Place all ingredients into a 6-8 quart pot with a tight fitting lid.

2. Cover with water and continue filling the pot until almost full. Put a tight-fitting lid on the pot. Bring to a boil (this takes about 10-20 minutes) then reduce the heat under the pot until the liquid is just simmering.

3. When the internal temperature of the chicken reaches 185 F remove it from the pot and leave it to cool down a bit (about 1 hour). Once the meat has been removed from the carcass put the bones back into the pot and continue simmering. You can also add any chicken bones that have been saved in the freezer for broth making. Refrigerate the chicken meat after it has cooled.

4. Keep the soup pot covered to prevent the stock from evaporating. Regardless the level will go down and you will probably have to add a few cups of water as the day progresses if you notice the liquid reducing too much.

5. When the broth has simmered and reduced to your satisfaction strain it through a fine mesh sieve. Discard the mushy veggies &and bones.

6. Cool stock and ladle into clean glass jars. The stock can be refrigerated for up to 3 days and will be fine in the freezer for up to 6 months.

Yield: About 4 quarts (16 one cup servings)

If using a slow cooker ... follow the steps outlined above. The chicken will likely take 2 ½-3 hours to reach an internal temperature of 185 F in the crock pot but it may take longer. (Crock pots vary in size and temperature). Remove meat from bones and return carcass to the pot and simmer from 4-24 hours.

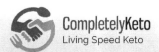

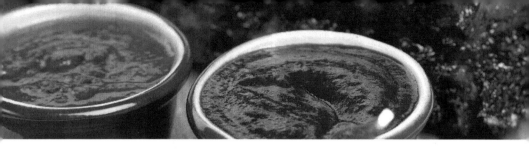

Smoky BBQ Sauce

This smoky BBQ sauce adds extra flavor to many different dishes plus it's totally Keto. I am especially fond of this sauce with baby back ribs and, of course, wings. So ... fire up the BBQ and enjoy!

Ingredients

- 2 T Coconut oil
- 1 medium Onion, fine dice
- 2 cloves Raw garlic, minced
- 2 T chili powder
- ½ tsp Black Pepper, ground
- ½ tsp Cumin, ground
- ½ tsp oregano, dried
- 1 T Basil, dried
- ¼ tsp Liquid Smoke
- 1 T Dijon Mustard
- 2 C Marinara Sauce, no sugar
- 2/3 C Vinegar, Apple Cider
- ¼ C water
- 1 tsp Hot Sauce, if desired
- 2/3 C Erythritol Sweetener (Zero Carb)

Preparation

1. Melt coconut oil in a stainless steel pot; add diced onion and sauté for a few minutes until softened.

2. Add minced garlic, chili powder, pepper, cumin, oregano and basil. Continue to sauté for another few minutes.

3. Add remaining ingredients and simmer, stirring occasionally, for 20 minutes.

Yield: approximately 2 cups (2 T/ serving)

Nutritional Information:

- Total Calories/serving: 41
- Total Carbs :4 g
- Fiber: 1 g
- Total Fat: 3 g
- Protein: 1 g

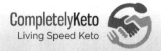

CompletelyKeto
Living Speed Keto

Breakfast Recipes

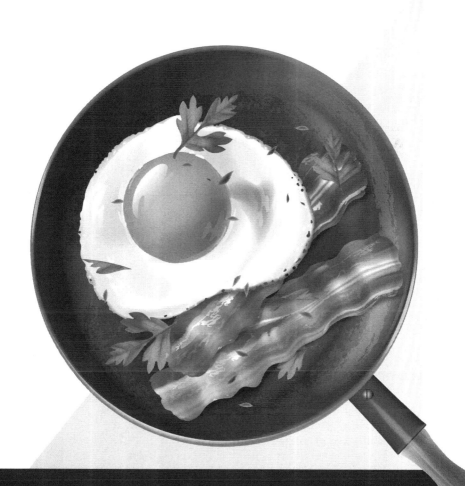

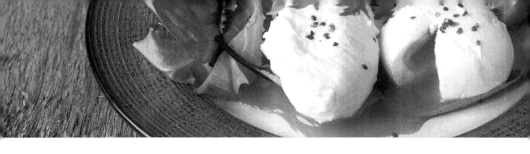

Perfectly Poached Eggs

It takes 4 minutes to perfectly poach one egg in water that is just at the simmering point. The end result is a nicely shaped egg with a warm yolk that is slightly thickened; not too runny or overly hard. Since we'll be poaching 4 eggs we will add about 20 seconds per extra egg. Some folks add a wee bit of vinegar to the simmering water which helps keep those wisps of egg white from escaping each egg and messing up the water. It takes practice to get perfectly poached eggs but is not impossible!

Ingredients

- 4 large eggs

Preparation

1. Select a pan, large enough to hold 4 eggs without them being too crowded, and fill it halfway up with water. Place pan over high heat and bring the water up to the boil. Reduce heat beneath the pan so the water is just at the simmering point. You will see small bubbles forming across the bottom of the pan that rise gently to the surface when the water is at the right temperature.

2. Crack fresh eggs, one at a time, into a measuring cup that has a long handle. Gently slip the eggs into the simmering water, one at a time. Poach the eggs for 5 minutes altogether.

3. Use a slotted spoon to remove each egg from the pan. I like to remove excess water by gently blotting the egg while it's still in the spoon. Serve while hot with a quick grinding of salt & pepper if desired.

Yield: Serves 4

Nutritional Information:

- Total Calories/serving: 70 (one egg/serving)
- Total Carbs: 0 g
- Fiber: 0 g
- Total Fat: 0 g
- Protein: 6 g

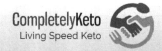
CompletelyKeto
Living Speed Keto

Keto Eggs Benny

Perfect for Sunday morning our Eggs Benny, keto style, is worth the extra bit of effort required. We employ a keto pancake in place of the English muffin that's used as a base in the traditional version. Replace the baked ham with turkey bacon or smoked chicken if pork isn't on your menu.

Ingredients

- 4 oz deli ham (or cooked turkey bacon/smoked chicken slice)
- 4 Keto Bread/Buns/Pancakes! (see recipe)
- 4 Perfectly Poached Eggs (see recipe)

For the Hollandaise sauce:

- 2 egg yolks
- Pinch of pink Himalayan salt
- Pinch of white pepper
- ¼ tsp powdered mustard
- ¼ C hot melted ghee

Preparation

1. Prepare the Keto pancakes ahead of time and have them ready to assemble the Eggs Benny when the time comes.

2. To make the Hollandaise sauce place egg yolks, salt, pepper and mustard powder in a blender and process on high until light and frothy.

3. Melt ghee. It must be liquid and hot for the next step.

4. Slowly drizzle the ghee into the blender while it is running at a higher speed. The yolk mixture will thicken into a sauce as you slowly drizzle in the hot ghee. Set sauce aside and keep warm while you poach the eggs.

5. Poach 4 eggs by following my directions for Perfectly Poached Eggs. (see recipe)

6. Assemble the Eggs Benny by placing a ham slice on top of each Keto Pancake. Put the hot poached egg on top and spoon some of the Hollandaise sauce on top of each poached egg. Garnish with a sprinkle of paprika and a bit of fresh parsley, if desired. Serve immediately while still hot.

Yield: Serves 4

Nutritional Information:

- Total Calories/serving: 713
- Total Carbs: 1 g
- Fiber: 0 g
- Total Fat: 26 g
- Protein: 14 g

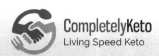

CompletelyKeto
Living Speed Keto

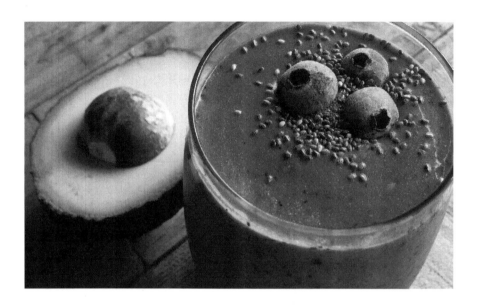

Blueberry Avocado Smoothie

Make a smoothie on a busy morning. You'll be out the door in no time!

Ingredients

- 1 C baby spinach leaves
- 1 ripe avocado
- 1 ½ C canned full fat coconut milk
- 1 T fresh lemon juice
- 1 tsp pure vanilla extract
- Allowed sweetener, to taste
- ½ C ice cubes

Preparation

1. Place all ingredients in blender and process on high speed until smooth. Divide equally between two glasses and serve.

Yield: Serves 2

Nutritional Information:

- Total Calories/serving: 166
- Total Carbs: 8 g
- Fiber: 5 g
- Total Fat: 15 g
- Protein: 2 g

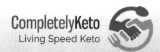
CompletelyKeto
Living Speed Keto

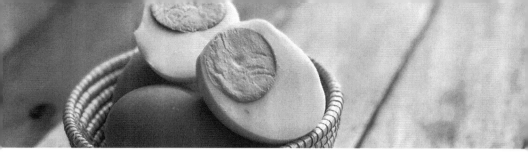

Perfectly Boiled Eggs

Keep a stash of ready to eat hard boiled eggs in the fridge for a quick snack if the need arises. I make boiled eggs using large sized eggs that come straight out of the fridge. Simply place eggs in a heavy bottomed pot that comfortably fits the number of eggs you are boiling. Cover the eggs with water (1" above the tops of the eggs in the pot) using cold water from the kitchen tap.

Hard Boiled Eggs:

Set your timer for 15 minutes and place the pot over high heat until the water boils. Immediately lower the heat to medium high so the water continues to boil but not at a rapid a rate.

When 15 minutes is up remove from heat and plunge the boiled eggs into ice cold water to immediately stop the cooking process. Refrigerate the eggs when cool enough to handle. Hard boiled eggs can be stored in the fridge for up to a week.

Soft Boiled Eggs:

Set your timer for 7 minutes and place the pot over high heat until the water boils. Immediately lower the heat to medium high so the water continues to boil but not at a rapid a rate.

When 7 minutes is up remove from heat and plunge the boiled eggs into ice cold water to immediately stop the cooking process. Take the top off the egg or peel and serve with ghee to add some saturated fat to your breakfast. Season with salt and pepper to taste.

Yield: 1 large egg per serving

Nutritional Information:

- Total Calories/serving: 70
- Total Carbs: 0 g
- Fiber: 0 g
- Total Fat: 2 g
- Protein: 6 g

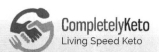

CompletelyKeto
Living Speed Keto

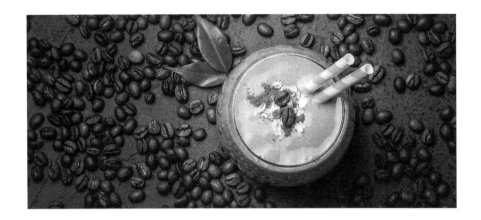

Mocha Smoothie

A breakfast smoothie is perfect for busy mornings when you need breakfast on the run or something easy for the morning commute. You can also add your daily dose of MCT oil into the mix and skip the Bullet Proof Coffee ritual if that makes your morning work better!

Ingredients

- 8 ice cubes, made with espresso or other strong coffee
- 2 C unsweetened coconut milk
- ½ tsp pure vanilla extract
- 1 T cocoa powder
- 1 avocado
- Allowed sweetener of choice, to taste

Preparation

1. Make coffee ice cubes the night before. I like to keep a bag of these ice cubes ready in the freezer.
2. Place all ingredients in blender and process on high speed until smooth. Divide equally between two glasses and serve.

Yield: Serves 2

Nutritional Information:

- Total Calories/serving 174
- Total Carbs: 9 g
- Fiber: 7 g
- Total Fat: 15 g
- Protein: 2 g

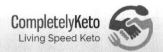

CompletelyKeto
Living Speed Keto

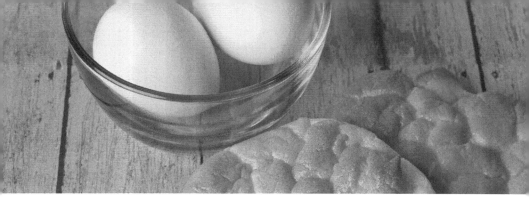

Keto Bread/Bun/Pancake!

Variations of a keto friendly Oopsie Bread or Cloud Bread abound on the internet with most recipes for this bread alternative using cream cheese. We like a version that uses mayonnaise instead of cream cheese making the end result perfect for our Speed Keto clients! Don't worry if you are making pancakes ... you won't taste the mayo!

Ingredients

- 3 large eggs, separated
- 3 T mayonnaise, full fat
- ½ tsp vanilla (if making pancakes)
- Few drops of liquid stevia or a pinch of the powder version, (if making pancakes)

Preparation

1. Pre-heat the oven to 350 F.
2. Whip egg whites until stiff
3. Beat egg yolks until light and creamy. Whisk in mayonnaise.
4. Carefully fold the egg yolk/ mayonnaise mixture into the egg whites.
5. Create 6 pancake shapes by mounding the mixture on a parchment lined baking sheet. (Make oval shaped pancakes if you are making buns for hot dogs). Bake on the middle rack of the pre-heated oven for 15 minutes. Cool on a wire rack.

Yield: serves 6 (one bun per serving)

Nutritional Information:

- Total Calories/serving: 80
- Total Carbs: 1 g
- Fiber: 0 g
- Total Fat: 8 g
- Protein: 3 g

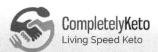

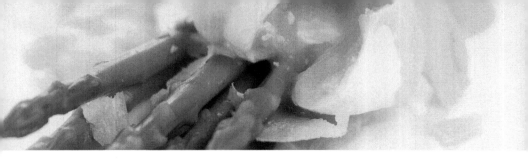

Poached Egg with Hollandaise on Asparagus

Ingredients

- 24 asparagus spears, washed and trimmed
- 4 large eggs

For the Hollandaise sauce:

- 2 egg yolks
- Pinch of pink Himalayan salt
- Pinch of white pepper
- ¼ tsp powdered mustard
- ¼ C hot melted ghee

Preparation

1. Place asparagus spears in a steamer basket over boiling water and steam until tender but still slightly crisp. The asparagus should be a nice bright green color. Keep warm until ready to use. Make the Hollandaise while the spears are in the steamer.

2. To make the Hollandaise sauce place egg yolks, salt, pepper and mustard powder in a blender and process on high until light and frothy. Melt ghee. It must be liquid and hot for the next step. Slowly drizzle the ghee into the blender while it is running at a higher speed. The yolk mixture will thicken into a sauce as you slowly drizzle in the hot ghee. Set sauce aside and keep warm while you poach the eggs.

3. Poach 4 eggs by following our recipe for Perfectly Poached Eggs. (see recipe)

4. Place an egg on 6 spears of steamed asparagus and garnish with a dollop of Hollandaise. Repeat with remaining ingredients. Serve immediately.

Yield: Serves 4

Nutritional Information:

- Total Calories/serving: 253
- Total Carbs: 4 g
- Fiber: 2 g
- Total Fat: 22 g
- Protein: 9

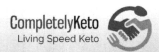
CompletelyKeto
Living Speed Keto

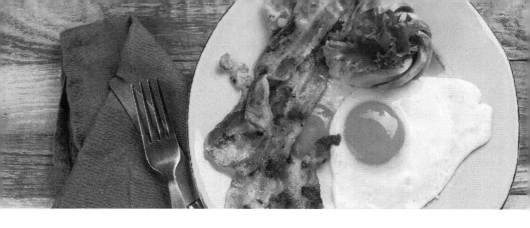

Bacon & Eggs

I like to include avocado on my breakfast plate occasionally to up the fat content. It also compliments the egg and salty turkey bacon flavors beautifully. Use regular bacon if that's your preference. Macros are provided at the end of this recipe for this breakfast both with and without the avocado.

Ingredients

- 2 bacon strips
- 1 large egg
- ½ ripe Hass avocado, thinly sliced

Preparation

1. Fry bacon until crisp and cooked through in a heavy bottomed skillet over medium high heat. Remove & drain on paper towel. Set aside and keep warm.

2. Fry egg in the hot bacon grease to your liking.

3. Serve with sliced avocado on the side if desired.

Yield: 1 serving

Nutritional Information:

- Total Calories/Serving (with avocado): 270
- Total Carbs: 8 g
- Fiber: 5 g
- Total Fat: 23 g
- Protein: 12
- Total Calories/Serving (no avocado): 150
- Total Carbs: 2 g
- Fiber: 0 g
- Total Fat: 12 g
- Protein: 11

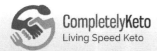

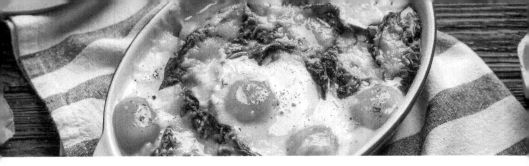

Baked Eggs Florentine

Ingredients

- 1 T ghee
- ½ small onion, fine dice
- 2 garlic cloves, peeled and pushed through a press
- 3 C baby spinach leaves
- 2 T coconut milk
- 1 T nutritional yeast
- 2 large eggs

Preparation

1. Pre-heat oven to 375 F.

2. Heat ghee over medium high heat. Add onion and sauté for 2 minutes. Add minced garlic and continue sautéing for 2 more minutes.

3. Stir in baby spinach leaves and sauté as the spinach wilts into the sautéed onion and garlic. Add the coconut milk and nutritional yeast and stir until the mixture is heated through.

4. Spray two small (individual portion size) casserole dishes with cooking oil and spread the spinach mixture across the bottom of the dish. Use a spatula to create a circular well or depressions in the centre of the spinach mixture. Crack the eggs into these depressions and grind some pink Himalayan salt and pepper over top.

5. Place the casseroles on the middle rack of the pre-heated oven and bake for 20 minutes, uncovered, or until the eggs are set and cooked to your liking. Serve immediately.

Yield: Serves 2

Nutritional Information:

- Total Calories/serving: 166
- Total Carbs: 5 g
- Fiber: 1 g
- Total Fat: 13 g
- Protein: 8 g

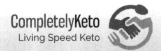

CompletelyKeto
Living Speed Keto

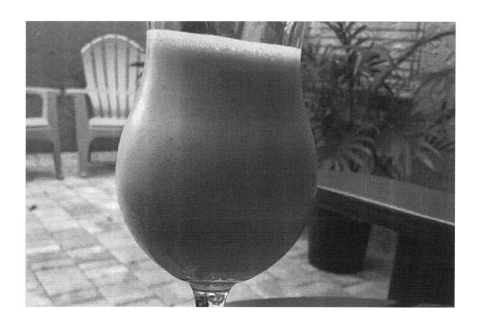

Chana Kilstein's Speed Keto Thick Shake

Thick, creamy and easy to whip up ...
Chana's breakfast shake is hard to beat.

Ingredients

- ½ C full fat coconut cream
- 2 T tahini
- 1/8 tsp cinnamon
- 8 – 12 ice cubes
- 1 2 droppers Sweet Leaf liquid stevia

Preparation

1. Add all ingredients to blender and process on high until thick and creamy.

Yield: Serves 2

Nutritional Information:

- Total Calories/serving: 163
- Total Carbs: 3 g
- Fiber: 1 g
- Total Fat: 14 g
- Protein: 3 g

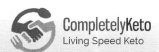

CompletelyKeto
Living Speed Keto

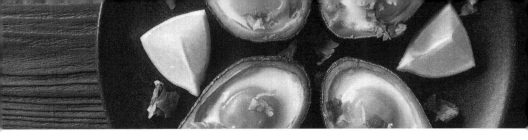

Baked Eggs in Avocado with Smoked Salmon

These eggs are perfect for a brunch with family and friends. They look elegant, plus they're easy to make. For a successful outcome you need to plan ahead so the avocados are ripe, but still firm, on the day you want to serve this dish.

Ingredients

- 2 ripe avocados, cut in halves and pits removed
- 3 oz smoked salmon, thinly sliced
- 4 Eggs
- Pinch of cayenne pepper
- 1 tsp pink Himalayan salt
- ¼ tsp ground black pepper corns
- Fresh herbs for garnish if desired
- Lemon wedges, for garnish if desired

Preparation

1. Preheat oven to 375 F
2. Cut avocados in half and remove the pits. Place, facing up with the peel side down, on a parchment lined baking sheet.
3. Crack one egg at a time into each avocado half place a thin slice of smoked salmon beside each egg inside the avocado depression.
4. Sprinkle salt, black pepper and cayenne evenly over the top of each egg.
5. Bake on the middle rack of the pre-heated oven for 20-25 minutes.
6. Garnish with freshly chopped herb of your choice. Place a lemon wedge on the side and serve immediately.

Yield: Serves 4

Nutritional Information:

- Total Calories/serving: 214
- Total Carbs: 6 g
- Fiber: 5 g
- Total Fat: 16 g
- Protein: 12 g

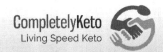

CompletelyKeto
Living Speed Keto

Lunch Recipes

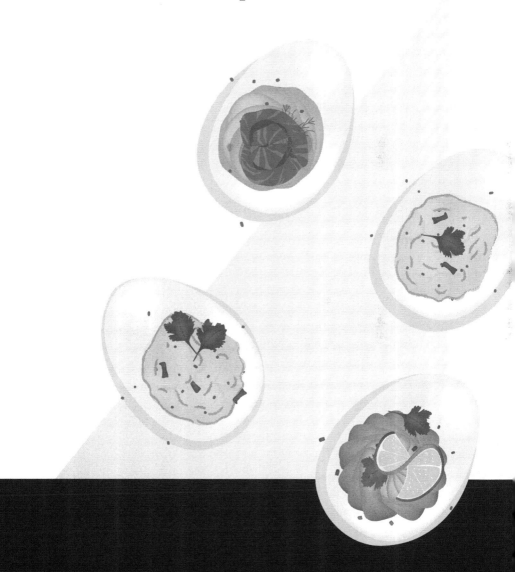

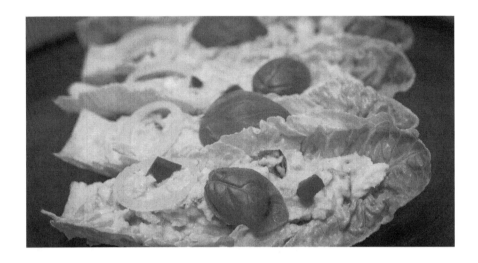

Tuna Salad on Romaine

Ingredients

- 1 can solid white tuna
- ¼ C full fat mayonnaise
- 8 Romaine lettuce leaves
- 2 onion slices
- ½ red bell pepper, small dice
- ¼ C baby spinach leaves
- Grinding of pink Himalayan salt & black pepper

Preparation

1. Place tuna in a small bowl. Use a fork to break up the tuna into smaller chucks. Add the mayo and stir until all the tuna is coated.

2. Place Romaine leaves on a platter and divide the tuna evenly between all the leaves.

3. Sprinkle diced red pepper over-top of the tuna and garnish with onion rings and spinach leaves. Serve immediately.

Yield: Serves 2

Nutritional Information:

- Total Calories/serving: 340
- Total Carbs: 6 g
- Fiber: 3 g
- Total Fat: 25 g
- Protein: 22 g

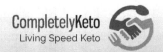
CompletelyKeto
Living Speed Keto

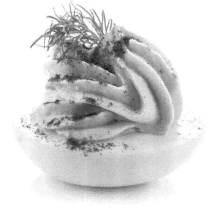
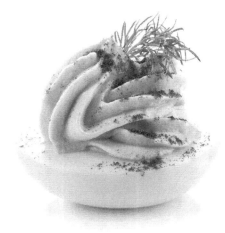

Curried Deviled Eggs

Deviled eggs never go out of style. We grew up eating them and so did our grandmothers. We've changed the recipe up by adding a bit of curry however let your taste buds guide you. If you prefer the traditional flavoring then leave the curry out! Serve dressed up with a slice of cucumber for an elegant appetizer at your next party.

Ingredients

- 2 large eggs, hard boiled
- 1 T full fat mayonnaise
- 1 tsp Dijon mustard
- ½ tsp onion powder
- ½ tsp curry powder
- Salt & pepper to taste
- 2 English cucumber slices, cut in half

Preparation

1. Cut hard boiled eggs in half lengthwise. Remove yolks and place them into a small bowl.

2. Add the mayo, Dijon mustard, onion powder and curry. Mash everything together using a fork and season to taste with salt & pepper.

3. Using a teaspoon carefully mound the yolk mixture into the egg halves. Garnish each with half cucumber slice and serve or refrigerate immediately.

Yield: 2 servings

Nutritional Information:

- Calories/serving: 118
- Total Carbs: 1 g
- Fiber: 0 g
- Total Fat: 10 g
- Protein: 6 g

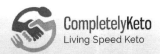

CompletelyKeto
Living Speed Keto

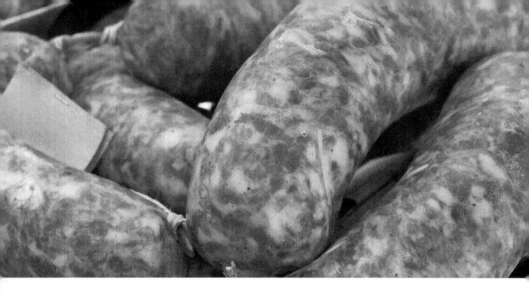

Italian Wedding Soup ... The Keto Version

This ketogenic version of traditional Italian Wedding Soup is high on our list of preferred comfort foods. We don't miss the tiny round pasta that's usually found in this soup and are very happy with the cauliflower "rice" we've substituted. Once the soup simmers in the pot for a while the cauliflower bits soften up as they absorb the broth and sausage flavors, providing a nice thickening element in our keto-friendly recipe.

Ingredients

- ½ C cooking onion, medium dice
- 1 T ghee or extra-virgin olive oil
- 1 C cauliflower florets (not frozen)
- 3 C chicken stock or bouillon
- 3 Italian Sausages
- 3 C baby spinach

Preparation

1. Sauté cooking onion over medium heat until soft and translucent.

2. Grate the cauliflower using a small food processor or box grater I to rice-sized bits and add to the pot.

3. Pour in the chicken broth and raise the heat under the pot until it begins to simmer. Adjust the heat so it continues to simmer.

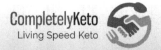

CompletelyKeto
Living Speed Keto

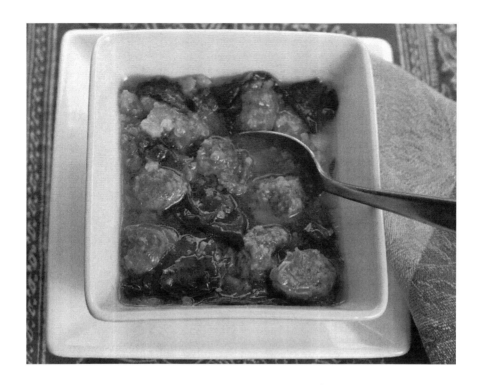

Italian Wedding Soup ... The Keto Version (continued)

4. Using sharp kitchen scissors snip the Italian sausages into tiny-sized meatball pieces. Add to the pot and continue to simmer for 15 minutes.

5. When you are ready to serve the soup stir in the baby spinach. It will quickly wilt into the broth. Remove the pot from the heat when the spinach is cooked but still a nice bright green. This will only take one or two minutes.

Yield: serves 3 (3 lunches on Speed Keto)

Nutritional Information:

- Calories/ serving: 344
- Total Carbs: 8 g
- Fiber: 2 g
- Total Fat: 27 g
- Protein: 17 g

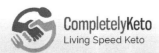

CompletelyKeto
Living Speed Keto

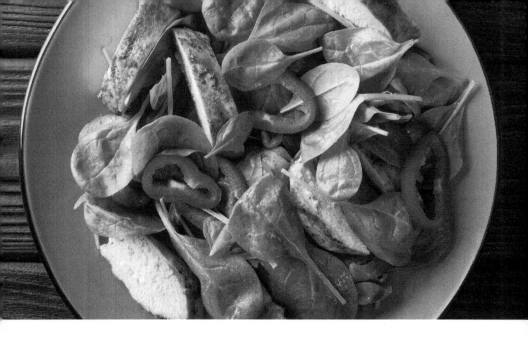

Spinach Salad with Chicken

Ingredients

- 4 C baby spinach leaves
- ½ C cooked chicken (grilled chicken breast)
- ½ red bell pepper
- 2 T red onion, minced
- 2 hard boiled eggs, mashed with a fork
- 2 bacon slices, cooked and crumbled (use either pork or turkey bacon)

Preparation

1. Divide spinach between salad bowls and top with chicken, pepper, onion, eggs and crumbled bacon
2. Drizzle your favorite allowed salad dressing over-top and enjoy!

Yield: Serves 2

Nutritional Information:

- Total Calories/serving: 260
- Total Carbs: 2 g
- Fiber: 0 g
- Total Fat: 12 g
- Protein: 36 g

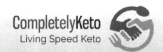

CompletelyKeto
Living Speed Keto

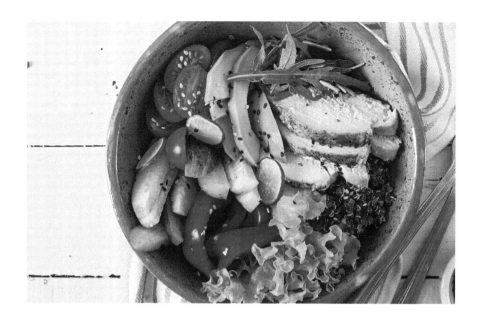

Turkey Buddha Lunch Bowl

Ingredients

- 4 C mixed greens
- 3 oz baked turkey breast (or use left-over turkey)
- 4 cherry tomatoes
- ½ Hass avocado, thin lengthwise slices
- ½ Red Bell Pepper, seeded and cut into strips
- ¼ English cucumber, cut into thin spears
- ¼ C Vinaigrette (see recipe)

Preparation

1. Divide mixed greens between two salad bowls
2. Evenly distribute the turkey breast slices, tomatoes, avocado, pepper and cucumber between both of the salads.
3. Drizzle 2 T of vinaigrette over each salad and serve.

Yield: Serves 2

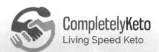

CompletelyKeto
Living Speed Keto

Old Fashioned Chicken Noodle Soup

This comforting chicken soup is made with konjac noodles making it completely keto. Konjac noodles are also known as yam noodles because they are made from a tuber which looks like a yam. Marketed as "Miracle" noodles, they contain zero carbs!

Ingredients

- 1 T extra virgin olive oil or coconut oil
- 1 yellow cooking onion, small dice
- ½ celery, small dice
- 1 tsp poultry seasoning
- 1 C shredded cabbage
- 1 quart box of organic chicken broth
- 4 – chicken leg/thigh quarters
- 1 package Konjac (also known as Yam or "Miracle") noodles

Preparation

1. Heat oil in a heavy bottomed soup pot.
2. Add diced onions and celery and poultry seasoning. Sauté until onions are translucent and the celery is soft.
3. Pour in the chicken broth and add the shredded cabbage and chicken quarters. Adjust the heat under the pot until the liquid is simmering nicely and allow the contents of the pot to simmer for about 40 minutes or until the internal temperature of the chicken reaches 165 F.
4. Take the chicken from the pot and allow it to cool until it can be easily handled. Remove the skin and discard. Take all the chicken from the bones and discard the bones. Drain and rinse the konjac noodles and add them to the contents of the pot along with the chicken.
5. Bring everything back up to the simmering point and continue simmering for 5 minutes. Serve when hot.

Nutritional Information:

- Total Calories/serving: 194
- Total Carbs: 5g
- Fiber: 1 g
- Total Fat: 14 g
- Protein: 13 g

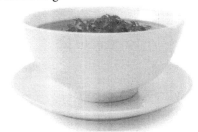

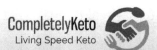

CompletelyKeto
Living Speed Keto

Dinner Recipes

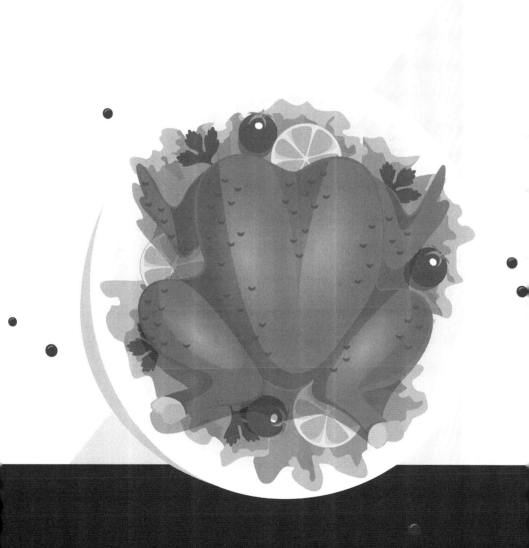

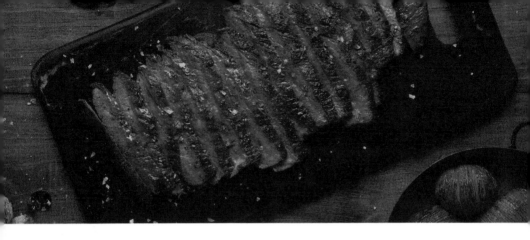

Flank Steak with Asian Slaw

Economical flank steak is perfect for this Asian flavored dish. The steak can be grilled on the BBQ if the weather is co-operating or you can simply use a heavy bottomed grill pan on your stove top to get the job done.

Ingredients

For the steak:

- 1/3 C extra-virgin olive oil
- 1 tsp dark sesame oil
- 2 garlic cloves, minced or pushed through a press
- 2 T apple cider vinegar
- 1/3 C wheat-free soy sauce (tamari)
- 2 tsp allowed sweetener of choice
- 1 ½ lb flank steak

For the Asian slaw:

- 2 tbsp wheat-free tamari soy sauce
- 2 tsp sambal oelek or sriracha sauce (hot sauce made without sugar)
- 1 tbsp fresh lemon or lime juice
- ½ C red onion, thinly sliced
- ½ lb cremini mushrooms
- 2 small bok choy or similar amount of a different type of Asian cabbage (about 2 C shredded)

For the sauce:

- ½ C full fat mayonnaise
- 1 tsp dark sesame oil (from toasted seeds)
- 1 tsp. allowed sweetener of your choice

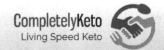

CompletelyKeto
Living Speed Keto

Preparation

1. Make a marinade by whisking the olive oil, sesame oil, garlic, vinegar, soy sauce and sweetener. Place flank steak in a large re-sealable plastic bag and pour the marinade over-top. Seal the bag and smoosh the marinade around inside the bag to coat the steak. Place the steak in the fridge for at least 2 hours before grilling. Flip the bag occasionally while it's resting in the fridge.

2. Make the Asian slaw by whisking soy sauce, hot sauce and vinegar in a bowl. Clean the onion and mushrooms then slice them all very thinly. Shred the cabbage lengthwise. Toss veggies with the dressing and set aside. Refrigerate if you make this earlier in the day.

3. To make the sauce mix the listed ingredients together. Set aside. Refrigerate if you make this earlier in the day. Remove from fridge and allow to come to room temperature before serving on top of the steak.

4. Remove meat from marinade, leaving some of the marinade on the meat so it won't stick to the pan or grill. Fry, in a preheated grill pan on the stove-top or grill on the BBQ over medium high heat for as long as it takes, depending on how you like your meat — medium rare or well done. Use a meat thermometer to check the internal temperature of the steak for best results; 120 F for rare or 130 F for medium-rare. The steak should rest, off the heat for 3 or 4 minutes before slicing. During this time the internal temperature will rise about 5 more degrees.

5. Slice into thin slanted pieces and fan the meat slices out on each plate.

6. Serve the meat with the Asian Slaw and a generous dollop of the sesame mayo sauce.

Serves 6

Nutritional Information:

- Total Calories/serving: 475
- Total Carbs: 5 g
- Fiber: 1 g
- Total Fat: 38 g
- Protein: 29 g

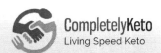

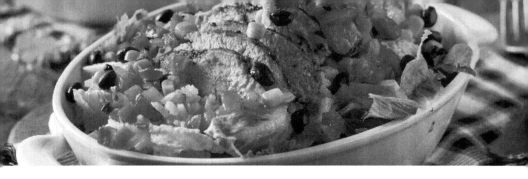

Fiesta Chicken Bowl

If you made homemade chicken broth you probably have cooked chicken available in your freezer that can easily be thawed for this dish. If not, just grill a small chicken breast. This quick meal is perfect for a night you are busy and must eat on the fly.

Ingredients

- ¼ C rice cauliflower, cooked and chilled
- ½ C cooked chicken
- 2 C Romaine lettuce, torn leaves
- 3 cherry tomatoes, cut in half
- 2 black olives, pitted and chopped
- 1 T red onion, fine dice
- ¼ avocado, cut into thin slices
- ½ jalapeño, seeded and fine dice
- 1 tsp taco seasoning
- 1 T, fresh lime juice
- 1 T extra-virgin olive oil

Preparation

1. Layer ingredients into the bowl in the following order: chilled cauliflower rice, romaine lettuce, cherry tomatoes, black olives, avocado, chicken chunks and jalapeño.

2. Make a dressing by whisking lime or lemon juice, taco seasoning and olive oil. Drizzle dressing over the bowl and serve.

Yield: Serves 1

Nutritional Information:

- Total Calories/serving: 375
- Total Carbs: 11 g
- Fiber: 4 g
- Total Fat: 26 g
- Protein: 30 g

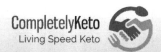
CompletelyKeto
Living Speed Keto

Stir-fried Pork & Broccoli

If you can, mix up the marinade and get the pork marinating at least 2 hours before you prepare this stir-fry. Serve on top of Konjac noodles (also known as Yam noodle or "Miracle Noodle) for a filling meal that done in a jiffy! Please substitute beef, turkey, or chicken if you do not eat pork.

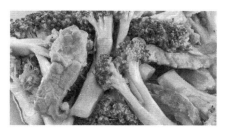

Ingredients

- 1 T extra-virgin olive oil
- 1 T fresh lemon juice
- ½ tsp oregano
- ½ lb pork tenderloin, cut into thin bite-sized strips
- 1 T coconut oil
- 1 C broccoli florets
- 1 or 2 packages of "Miracle" noodles

Preparation

1. Make the marinade by whisking the olive oil, fresh lemon juice and oregano.
2. Place the strips of pork tenderloin in a re-sealable plastic bag and pour the marinade over-top. Seal the bag and smoosh it around to ensure all the pork is covered. Refrigerate until ready to stir-fry.
3. Drain the pork and discard the left-over marinade.
4. Rinse miracle noodles, set aside.
5. Heat ½ T of ghee in the wok over medium high heat and add the pork strips.
6. Toss and stir-fry until the pork is evenly cooked, all the way through, This will take about 4 minutes. Remove from wok and keep warm. Wipe out the wok.
7. Cut broccoli florets into smaller florets if necessary, so they take less time to stir-fry. Melt coconut oil and add the broccoli. Stir fry until almost done and add the pork back into the wok. Continue to toss and stir-fry for 1 more minutes. Add the noodles, cover the wok and heat for one minute. Serve immediately.

Yield: Serves 2

Nutritional Information:

- Total Calories/serving: 199
- Total Carbs: 5 g
- Fiber: 1 g
- Total Fat: 9 g
- Protein: 24 g

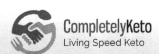
CompletelyKeto
Living Speed Keto

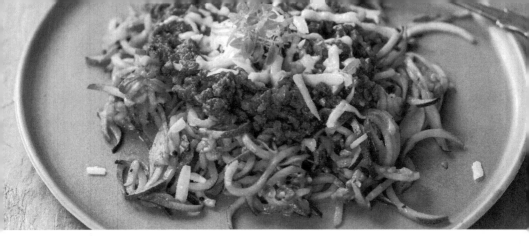

Spaghetti Bolognese

Our Spaghetti Bolognese is packed with flavor and doesn't take long to make. It's proven to be a client favorite and often receives positive comments on the website.

Ingredients

- ½ C cremini mushrooms, thin slices
- 1 ½ T extra-virgin olive oil or coconut oil
- ½ medium onion, small dice
- 3 garlic cloves, about 2 T minced
- 2 C ground beef
- 2 C unsweetened tomato sauce
- 2 tsp dried oregano
- 1 tsp dried basil
- ½ tsp salt
- ½ tsp ground black pepper
- 1 bay leaf
- 1 T ghee
- 2 small zucchini, about 6" in length

Preparation

1. Sauté mushrooms in olive oil over medium high heat until soft and cooked through. Remove from heat and set aside

2. In a separate skillet sauté diced onion for a few minutes in the remaining ½ T of olive oil. When onion is soft and translucent add half of the minced garlic and continue to sauté for one minute more.

3. Add ground beef to the skillet and turn the heat up to medium high. Continue stirring the beef as it sautés until it is nicely browned.

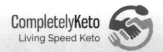
CompletelyKeto
Living Speed Keto

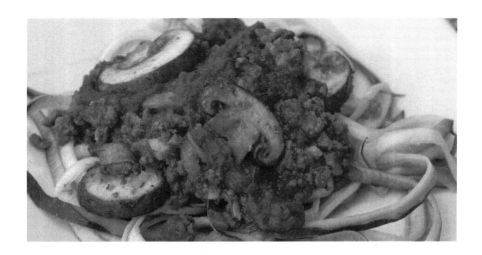

Spaghetti Bolognese (continued)

4. Mix in the tomato sauce, bay leaf, oregano, basil, cooked mushrooms, salt and pepper and lower the heat to medium low so the sauce is just simmering.

5. Wash zucchini, pat dry and trim the ends. Spiralize into noodles. You will have about 4 – 5 cups of "veggie pasta" when done. Chop the left-over zucchini core and stir it into the simmering Bolognese sauce. Continue simmering the sauce for another 5 minutes.

6. When it's time to serve the meal melt the ghee in a separate skillet and add the remaining minced garlic. Sauté for one minute over medium heat then add the spiral zucchini noodles. Continue to sauté until the noodles are somewhat wilted but still al dente in texture. This won't take long (about 1 ½ - 2 minutes). Divide into 4 portions. Serve with the Bolognese Sauce ladled over-top.

Yield: Serves 4

Nutritional Information

- Total Calories/serving: 231
- Total Carbs: 9 g
- Fiber: 3 g
- Total Fat: 16 g
- Protein: 14 g

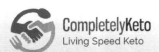

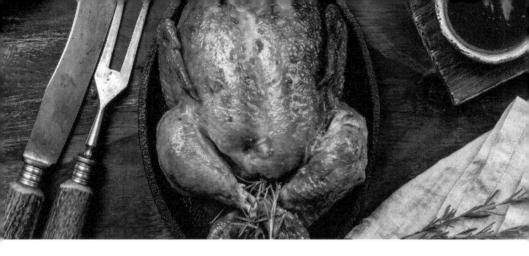

Simple Roast Chicken

Remember to save the carcass in the freezer after you've pulled all the meat from the bones. You can throw these bones in the soup pot the next time you're making Chicken broth. At the end of this recipe for Simple Roast Chicken I've included nutritional information for a number of different variations on this meal.

Ingredients

- 1 whole chicken
- ½ cooking onion, peeled
- 2 cloves garlic
- 1 T extra-virgin olive oil
- ½ tsp dried thyme
- ½ tsp dried oregano
- 2 C broccoli florets
- Salt & pepper

Preparation

1. Pre-heat oven to 500 F

2. Rinse chicken, inside and out with cool water and pat dry. Remove excess fat from around the edges of the chicken cavity then place the half onion and garlic cloves inside the cavity. Put the chicken into a roasting pan.

3. Brush outside of chicken with olive oil and sprinkle the thyme, oregano, salt and pepper over the skin surface. Place the pan on the middle rack of the pre-heated oven.

4. Immediately reduce the oven heat to 350 F and roast the chicken for about one hour. Baste the chicken with the pan drippings and return to the oven for about another ½ hr or until

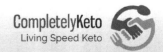

CompletelyKeto
Living Speed Keto

Simple Roast Chicken (continued)

the internal temperature reaches 165 F (test both white and dark meat areas). Let the chicken rest on a platter for 5 minutes while you prepare the broccoli.

5. Steam broccoli flowerets for 3-5 minutes until cooked but still a nice bright green color. Carve chicken and serve with steamed broccoli florets on the side.

Yield: Serves 4 (save some for lunch tomorrow)

Nutritional Information

(with ½ C steamed broccoli florets):

- Total Calories/serving: 312
- Total Carbs: 8 g
- Fiber: 2 g
- Total Fat: 16 g
- Protein: 30 g

Nutritional Information

(with Spinach & Garlic Side Dish - see recipe)

- Total Calories/serving: 285

- Total Carbs: 4 g
- Fiber:0 g
- Total Fat: 16 g
- Protein: 29 g

Nutritional Information

(with ¼ C spinach, 2 cherry tomatoes, 4 slices cucumber and a garlic dill pickle on the side)

- Total Calories/serving: 311
- Total Carbs: 10 g
- Fiber: 2 g
- Total Fat:17 g
- Protein: 30 g

Nutritional Information

(with 4 steamed asparagus spears/ serving)

- Total Calories/serving: 302
- Total Carbs: 7 g
- Fiber: 2 g
- Total Fat: 16 g
- Protein: 31 g

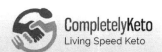

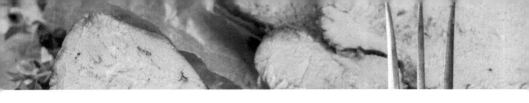

Roasted Turkey Breast

Don't wait for Thanksgiving or Christmas to enjoy a turkey dinner. Nowadays, turkey is available in cut up sections at most supermarkets and butcher shops. Roasted Turkey Breast is thrown together easily and will definitely be a family and friend pleaser.

Ingredients

- 2 ½ lb turkey breast, with skin
- 1 ½ T extra-virgin olive oil
- 1 T kosher salt
- 1 tsp dried thyme
- 1 tsp dried sage
- 1 tsp smoked paprika
- 1 tsp ground black pepper
- 8 garlic cloves
- 4 small shallots, peeled and cut in half
- 3 celery stalks, cut into chunks
- ½ bunch fresh flat-leaf parsley, chopped

Preparation

1. Pre-heat oven to 450 F.
2. Brush oil onto the turkey breast and season with salt, thyme, sage, paprika, and pepper.
3. Mix together the garlic cloves, celery stalks and chopped parsley. Make a pile in the bottom of a roasting pan and place the seasoned turkey breast on top of the veggies.
4. Place uncovered pan on the middle rack of the pre-heated oven and immediately turn the temperature down to 325 F.
5. Roast the breast, basting occasionally after the first hour for about 1 ½ hours in total. The internal temperature of the turkey breast should be 165 F when it is done. Serve turkey slices with the roasted veggies (from beneath the turkey breast) and a side salad.

Yield: Serves 6

Nutritional Information:

- Total Calories/serving: 205
- Total Carbs: 5 g
- Fiber: 4 g
- Total Fat: 5 g
- Protein: 32 g

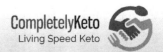

CompletelyKeto
Living Speed Keto

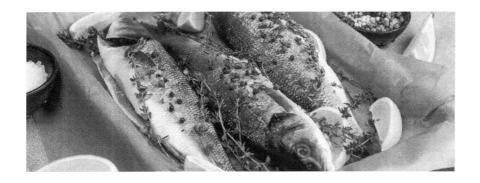

Baked Whole Fish; Thai Style

This recipe will work with any individual portion-sized whole fish; like trout, bream or sea bass. As is the case for most meat and fish, when cooked on the bone the resulting flavor is amplified. Cook fish whole, in foil packets, on the BBQ or bake in the oven. Simple yet elegant, whole fish make a stunning presentation on the plate.

Ingredients

- 4 whole fish – sea bass, trout or bream
- 4 plum tomatoes, cut into 3 or 4 slices each
- 4 lemon grass stalks, 4" pieces
- Grinding of pink Himalayan salt & black pepper
- 4 garlic cloves, cut into slivers

- 4 T minced chili pepper, select pepper with the level of heat you prefer
- 2 T minced fresh ginger

Preparation

1. Preheat oven to 350 F (or preheat the BBQ to medium high)
2. On the counter lay out 4 pieces of aluminum foil large enough to make a sealed packet around each of the whole fish.
3. Arrange 3 or 4 tomato slices in the center of each foil piece. Place whole fish on top of the tomato slices.
4. Insert lemon grass into the cavity of each fish. Grind salt and pepper over each fish and sprinkle the garlic, chili pepper and fresh ginger over top.

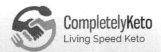

CompletelyKeto
Living Speed Keto

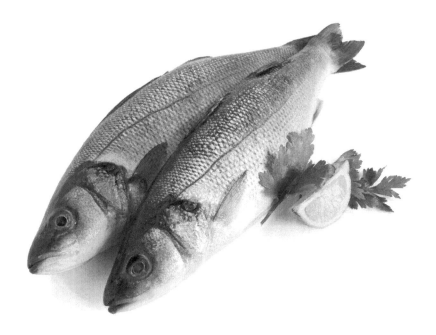

Baked Whole Fish; Thai Style (continued)

5. Wrap foil around the fish and seal the ends to form a tight packet.

6. Oven method: place fish packets on a large flat baking sheet and bake on the middle rack of the pre-heated oven for about 15 minutes or until the fish is flaky (but not dry) and cooked through.

7. BBQ method: Place fish packets on the BBQ and bake for 6 minutes on each side.

8. Serve with steamed veggies or and/or a salad of your choice on the side.

Yield: Serves 4

Nutritional Information:

- Total Calories/serving: 224
- Total Carbs: 11 g
- Fiber: 2 g
- Total Fat: 9 g
- Protein: 25 g

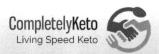

CompletelyKeto
Living Speed Keto

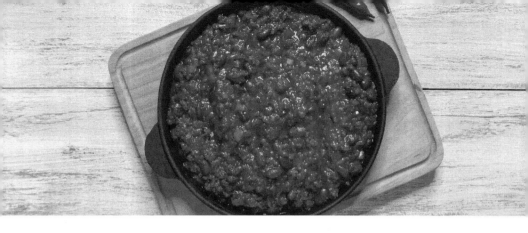

Keto Chili

The chili freezes well so you can double the recipe for easy meals. Make this completely keto chili with either ground beef or ground turkey. Pop what's left-over in the freezer for a quickly prepared meal when Keto Chili shows up in the menu plan again.

Ingredients

- 1 T extra virgin olive oil
- ½ cooking onion, medium dice
- 4 garlic cloves, minced or pushed through a press
- 1 lb ground beef or ground turkey
- ½ T chili powder
- ½ tsp ground cumin
- 1 tsp smoked chipotle powder
- 1 tsp pink Himalayan salt flakes
- ½ tsp black pepper
- 1 ½ C organic beef broth
- 2 C riced cauliflower
- 2 jalapeño peppers, seeded and minced finely (leave seeds in if you like heat!)
- 1 medium tomato, medium dice
- 2 T tomato paste
- ½ T sweetener, of choice
- ½ C fresh cilantro, finely chopped (large stems removed)
- 1 sprig fresh cilantro, for garnish

Preparation

1. Pre-heat oven to 325 F
2. Heat olive oil in a heavy, oven-proof pot over medium high heat. Add onion and sauté for 2 or 3 minutes. Add garlic and continue to sauté for 2 more minutes.

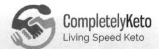

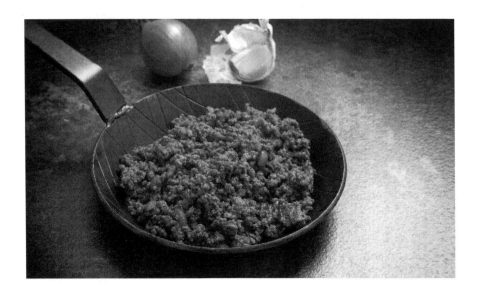

Keto Chili (continued)

3. Add ground beef to the skillet and sauté until the meat is almost browned. Add spices, salt and pepper and continue to sauté until the meat is nicely browned.

4. Stir in the stewed tomatoes, beef broth and tomato paste. Add the diced jalapeño and riced cauliflower and give the ingredients a good stir to incorporate all the ingredients. Bring to a boil. Remove from heat immediately, cover pot with a tight fitting lid and place on the middle rack of the pre-heated oven.

5. Bake for 2 hours, stirring occasionally until the meat is tender and the all the flavors are well developed. Serve while hot or cool and refrigerate. This recipe also freezes well.

Yield: Serves 6

Nutritional Information:

- Total Calories/serving: 217
- Total Carbs: 7 g
- Fiber: 2 g
- Total Fat: 14 g
- Protein: 18 g

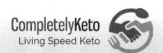

CompletelyKeto
Living Speed Keto

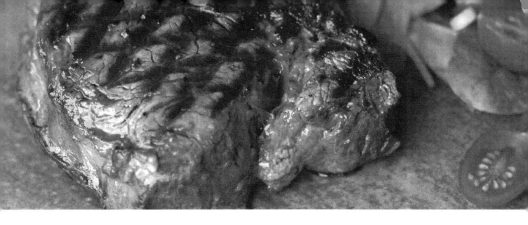

Perfect Steak

If you can afford it, treat yourself to a nicely marbled filet mignon steak. We also like the strip loin and T-bone beef cuts. Look for nice lines of fat running through the meat and try to get steaks that are at least 1 ½" thick for best results. Also, get yourself a decent digital meat thermometer if you don't already have one. This will ensure great results every time.

We like to keep it simple letting the taste of good beef shine through. Just a bit of salt & pepper and that's it; you are good to go!

Ingredients

- 4 filet mignon steaks, each 1 ½" thick and about 6 oz.
- Himalayan salt flakes
- freshly ground pepper

Preparation

1. Sprinkle salt flakes over each of the steaks followed by a grinding of fresh pepper. Flip the steaks and repeat.

2. BBQ Method: Pre-heat the grill to high and the sear the steaks for 2 minutes on each side with the lid open. Then lower the heat to medium, close the lid and continue grilling for 2 or 3 more minutes per side. The time will vary depending on the thickness of the steaks and your preference for "doneness". You will want to remove the steaks from the grill when the internal temperature reaches 120 F in the center for rare or 130 F for medium-rare. Let the steaks rest for a few minutes during which time the internal temp will rise about 5 more degrees.

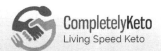

CompletelyKeto
Living Speed Keto

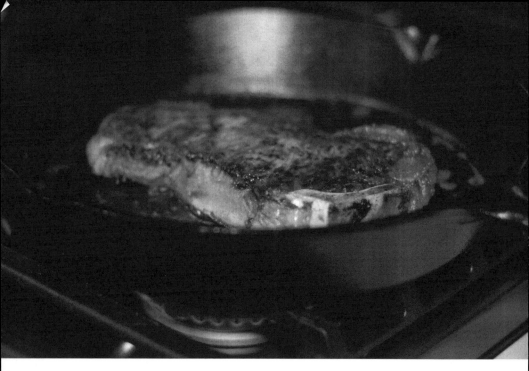

Perfect Steak (continued)

3. Stove-top Method: We use a cast-iron grill pan for steaks cooked on the stove top. Turn the element to high and let the pan, sprayed with cooking oil, get good and hot. Quickly sear the steaks on each side then turn the heat under the pan down to medium-high. Continue frying the steaks for 2 or 3 minutes per side. When the internal temperature reaches 120F – 130 F (as described above) remove from the pan and let rest for a few minutes before serving.

Yield: Serves 4

Nutritional Information:

- Total calories: 420
- Total Carbs: 0 g
- Fiber: 0 g
- Net Carbs: 0 g
- Total Fat: 30 g
- Protein: 34 g

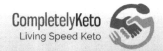

CompletelyKeto
Living Speed Keto

Harlan's Thai Red Curry Chicken Soup

Dinner in a bowl; fragrant, spicy and oh so yummy! Harlan struck it out of the ballpark with this one.

Ingredients

- 1 tsp extra virgin olive oil
- 1 small cooking onion, small dice
- 1 red bell pepper, thinly sliced
- 3 garlic cloves, minced or pushed through a press
- 3 T red curry paste
- 1 tsp fresh ginger root, minced
- 1 tsp turmeric
- 6 C organic chicken broth
- 1 can full fat coconut milk
- 2 C cooked chicken, shredded (use cooked chicken left-over from making broth or fry 2 chicken breasts & shred)
- 1 zucchini, spiralized
- Thin slices of lime and fresh cilantro leaves, for garnish

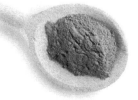

Preparation

1. Heat oil in a large, heavy bottomed pot over medium heat. Add onion and sauté for 2 minutes. Add pepper and continue to sauté for 2 more minute. Add garlic and sauté for one minute more.

2. Add red curry paste, ginger and turmeric to veggies. Stir until combined. Allow the spices to cook for 30 seconds the add the broth and coconut milk. Bring to the boil and adjust heat so liquid is just simmering. Simmer, uncovered, for 20 minutes. Add cooked chicken and continue simmering for 10 minutes.

3. Ladle into bowls and add zucchini noodles. Top with cilantro and lime slices. Serve with a Tsippy Roll on the side. (see recipe).

Yield: Serves 6

Nutritional Information:

- Total Calories/serving: 155
- Total Carbs: 7 g
- Fiber: 2 g
- Total Fat: 6 g
- Protein: 8 g

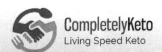

CompletelyKeto
Living Speed Keto

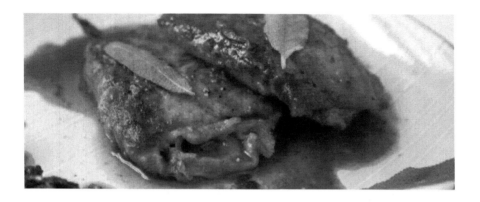

Harlan's Chicken Saltimbocca

Chicken breasts don't have to be dull. In this recipe, the chicken is paired with thin slices of pastrami and flavored with sage, garlic, lemon and wine. Chicken Saltimbocca is a keto classic that graces my table often.

Ingredients

- 2 lb chicken breasts, boneless & skinless
- 12 fresh sage leaves
- 2 C organic chicken stock
- 4 T extra virgin olive oil
- 3 T minced garlic
- 1 C Pinot Grigio
- ¼ lb navel Pastrami slices
- 1 ½ T fresh lemon juice
- Fresh basil for garnish

Preparation

1. Use a mallet or rolling pin to pound each chicken breast until flat and thin. Sprinkle with salt & pepper

2. Place one sage leaf over each slice of chicken and wrap a slice of pastrami over the chicken.

3. Heat a large skillet on high heat. When hot, drizzle half of the olive oil into the skillet. Place half of the Saltimbocca's into the skillet and sear on each side for about a minute or two. Remove from skillet and repeat with the remaining 4 pieces using rest of the olive oil. Place all on a plate and set on the side.

4. Add garlic and wine to the same skillet and place over medium-high heat. Using your spatula

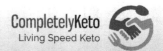
CompletelyKeto
Living Speed Keto

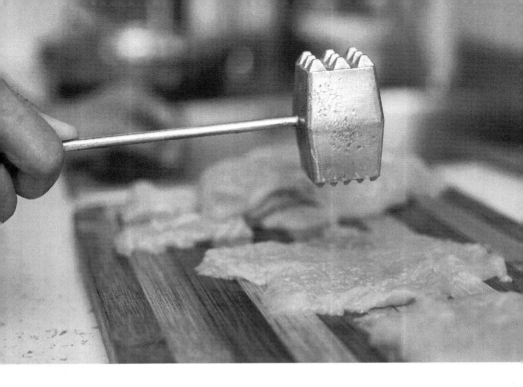

Harlan's Chicken Saltimbocca (continued)

gently rub off the brown bits stuck on the bottom of the skillet to incorporate into the wine mixture. Raise heat to high, and add zest of lemon, lemon juice and the rest of the sage leaves. Reduce heat to low. Simmer until wine is reduced by half.

5. Return all pieces of Saltimbocca to the skillet. Pour chicken stock into the skillet and simmer for 5 – 8 minutes over medium-high heat until reduced by half.

6. Remove the Saltimbocca's from the skillet and place on a platter. Garnish with fresh basil leaves. Serve immediately.

Yield: Serves 6

Nutritional Information:

- Total Calories/serving: 240
- Total Carbs: 5 g
- Fiber: 2 g
- Total Fat: 11 g
- Protein: 26 g

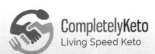

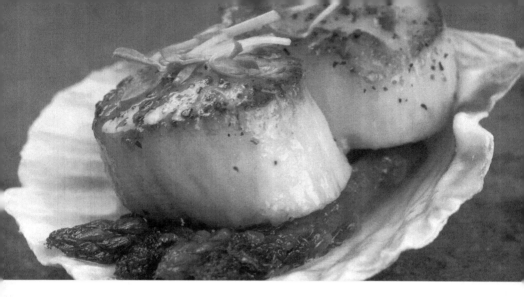

Seared Scallops on Sautéed Asparagus

I have to treat myself to large succulent scallops every once in awhile. This recipe does them justice and the bonus is; they don't take long to get onto the table.

Ingredients

- 3 T ghee (or extra virgin olive oil)
- 1 ½ lb large scallops
- 1 lb asparagus spears
- ½ tsp ground black pepper
- ½ tsp pink Himalayan salt
- ¼ C Pinot Grigio
- 1 tsp white wine vinegar
- 1 T coconut oil

Preparation

1. Heat 1 T of the ghee (or oil) in a large, heavy bottomed non-stick skillet over medium-high heat. Saute the asparagus, stirring occasionally until tender but still a bright green in color. This will take approximately 5 minutes. Transfer the asparagus spears to a plate and keep warm.

2. Add an additional T of ghee to the skillet and heat over medium high heat. Pat scallops dry and sprinkle with salt and pepper. Place half the scallops in the pre-heated pan. Make sure to leave some room between each scallop. This allows them to brown nicely. Flip the

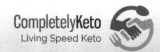

CompletelyKeto
Living Speed Keto

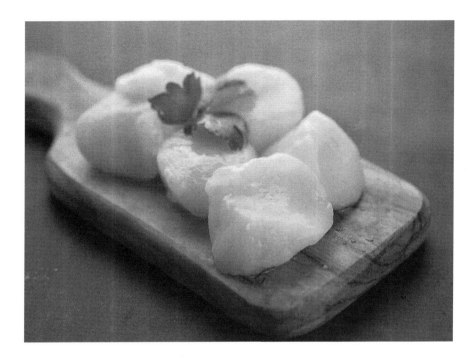

scallops over after 3 minutes and continue cooking for 2 more minutes or until the scallops are seared and browned on both sides. Transfer each scallop to a warm plate as they are done. Repeat this process with the remaining scallops.

3. Add the wine and vinegar to the skillet. Simmer while stirring to scrape the brown bits up off the bottom of the skillet. Reduce the liquid slightly then swirl in the coconut oil. When melted remove the sauce from the heat.

4. Divide asparagus spears between 6 warmed plates and top with scallops. Drizzle sauce over-top and serve immediately.

Yield: Serves 6

Nutritional Information:

- Total Calories/serving: 215
- Total Carbs: 8 g
- Fiber: 2 g
- Total Fat: 12 g
- Protein: 19 g

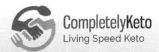

CompletelyKeto
Living Speed Keto

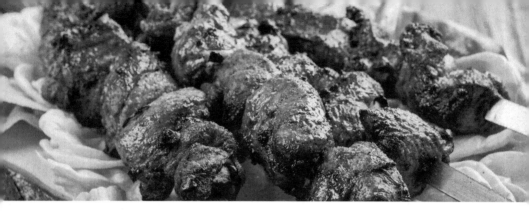

Lamb Souvlaki

Here's another easy meal for a busy night when you need to eat and run. If you can, cut up the lamb and get it into the marinade in the morning, before you head out the door.

Ingredients

- 1 ½ lbs boneless lamb shoulder
- ¼ C lemon juice
- 2 garlic cloves, minced or pushed through a press
- 2 tsp dried oregano
- ¼ C extra virgin olive oil
- ¼ tsp salt
- ¼ tsp pepper

Preparation

1. Cut lamb into 1" cubes and place in a re-sealable bag.
2. Mix together lemon juice, garlic, oregano and olive oil. Pour over lamb and seal bag. Refrigerate for at least an hour and up to 24 hours.
3. Thread lamb onto 8 skewers & place on a foil lined baking sheet. Discard the left-over marinade.
4. Broil 6 inches away from the heat for about 4 or 5 minutes per side. The internal temperature of the meat cubes should be 145 F when they are done. Serve immediately.

Yield: serves 4 (2 skewers per serving)

Nutritional Information:

- Total Calories/serving: 353
- Total Carbs: 2 g
- Fiber: 0 g
- Total Fat: 18 g
- Protein: 21 g

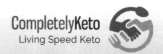

CompletelyKeto
Living Speed Keto

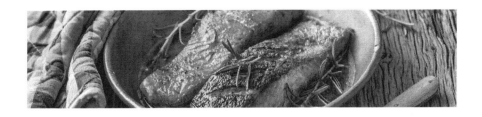

Crispy Skin Salmon Fillet

Key to getting a nice crisp on Salmon skin is preheating a heavy bottomed skillet before searing the fillet; preferably a cast iron skillet. Follow the directions below and you will have success every time!

Ingredients

- 1 T extra virgin olive oil or coconut oil
- 2-4oz salmon fillets
- Sprigs of rosemary and/or thyme

Preparation

1. Pre-heat oven to 350 F
2. Place heavy skillet or cast iron frying pan in oven while it's pre-heating to get the pan good and hot (this will result in nice crispy salmon skin on the bottom of the fillet)
3. Heat the oil up in the pre-heated skillet over medium high heat. You should here a sizzle/ popping sound when you put the fillets in the pan, however you don't want it so hot that the oil is smoking. Fry the fillets for 2-3 minutes, skin side down. Baste the top of the fillets with the hot oil.
4. Add sprigs of rosemary and thyme to the pan and transfer the skillet onto the middle rack of the pre-heated oven. Bake the salmon for about 4 more minutes or until the salmon is moist and just slightly flaky. The amount of time will depend on the thickness of the fillets. Serve immediately.

Yield: 2 servings

Nutritional Information:

- Total Calories/serving: 169
- Total Carbs: 0 g
- Fiber: 0 g
- Total Fat: 12 g
- Protein: 14 g

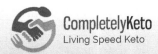
CompletelyKeto
Living Speed Keto

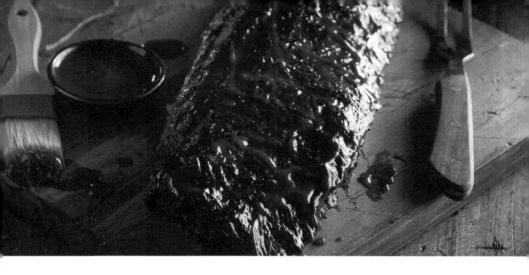

Oven Baked Baby Back Ribs

Ribs are still on the menu! We love them when basted with Harlan's Secret BBQ Sauce. Pair ribs with Mock Potato Salad for a picnic style meal, any time of the year!

Ingredients

For the rub:

- 1 T garlic powder
- 1 T onion powder
- 1 tsp allowed sweetener of choice
- 1 tsp pink Himalayan salt
- ½ tsp chili powder
- ½ tsp smoked chipotle powder
- ½ tsp paprika
- 1/8 tsp cumin

For the ribs:

- 1 T Dijon mustard
- 2 full racks of baby back spare ribs
- ½ C Smokey BBQ sauce (see recipe)

Preparation

1. Pre-heat the oven to 350 F.

2. Make the rub by mixing together the garlic powder, onion powder, sweetener, salt, chili powder, smoked chipotle powder, paprika & cumin. Set aside.

3. Prepare the ribs by removing the paper thin membrane from the backside of the rib bones. This membrane is almost invisible

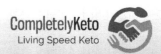
CompletelyKeto
Living Speed Keto

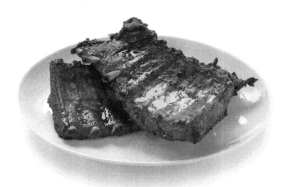

Oven Baked Baby Back Ribs (continued)

and it's hard to find. Once you manage to lift a corner here's a trick that will help you pull the membrane off. Using a small piece of paper towel, grip the loosened edge of the membrane and pull it away from the ribs. This will keep your fingers from slipping and the membrane should come off in one easy piece.

4. Cover two rimmed baking sheets with foil.

5. Coat the ribs (both front and back) with the mustard. Sprinkle the spice rub mixture, evenly, over both sides of the rack and arrange ribs on the baking sheets. Brush 2-3 T of BBQ sauce over-top each rack and place on the middle rack of the pre-heated oven. Bake for one hour, bon more BBQ sauce and return to oven.

6. Bake for another hour or until the internal temperature reaches 180-190 degrees F. Gauging the temperature of ribs using a thermometer is tricky but a visual check also works well. When ribs are done you can easily see how the meat pulls away from the edge of the rib bones, leaving about ¼" of bone showing along the side of the racks. When you see this has happened it indicates the fats and collagens have melted leaving you with a tender and tasty rack. Enjoy!

Yield: Serves 4 (1/2 rack per serving)

Nutritional Information:

- Total Calories/serving: 505
- Total Carbs: 7 g
- Fiber: 1 g
- Total Fat: 40 g
- Protein: 32 g

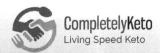

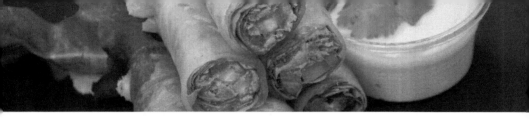

Tex/Mex Fish Roll-ups

These roll-ups work well for dinner or lunch. You can make them many different types of fish and even a can of tuna will do in a pinch!

Ingredients

- 2 T ghee
- Grinding of pink Himalayan salt & pepper
- ½ lb fish (cod, halibut, flounder, haddock)
- 1 tsp taco seasoning
- 1 medium tomato, small dice
- 4 scallions, thin slices
- 1 ripe avocado
- Boston Lettuce (or other leaf lettuce), you need 8 large leaves
- ½ C full fat mayonnaise
- 2 T freshly squeezed lemon juice

Preparation

1. Season the fish on both sides with a grinding of salt & pepper. Sprinkle on ½ tsp of the taco seasoning.
2. Melt ghee in a heavy bottomed skillet over medium high heat and fry the fish until done (about 5 minutes). Flip the fish about half way through the cooking process. Pull cooked fish apart into smaller chunks.
3. Make the sauce by whisking mayonnaise, lemon juice, remaining taco seasoning and dash of hot sauce.
4. Pull lettuce leaves apart. Wash & pat dry.
5. Divide fish, diced tomato, avocado & sliced scallions amongst the 8 lettuce leaves. Spoon on sauce. Fold sides of leaves inwards over to filling then starting on one edge, roll them up.

Yield: serves 4 (2 roll-ups/serving)

Nutritional Information:

- Total Calories/serving: 400
- Total Carbs: 9 g
- Fiber: 4 g
- Total Fat: 34 g
- Protein: 12 g

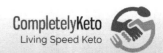
CompletelyKeto
Living Speed Keto

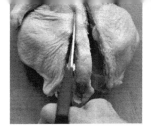
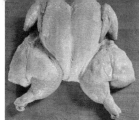
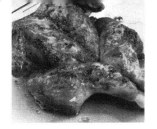

Roasted Spatchcocked Chicken

It's easy to Spatchcock a whole chicken. Use sharp poultry sheers to cut along either side of the chicken backbone:

Discard the backbone and flip the chicken over. Press down on the chicken firmly to flatten it out:

Now you are ready to roast this Spatchcocked chicken in the oven. When flattened out like this, chicken cooks a bit faster and the breasts are never dry. Tuck fresh herb sprigs, some garlic cloves and lemon slices beneath the chicken as it roasts for added delicate flavoring.

Ingredients

- 1 whole chicken (5 – 6 lbs)
- Herb sprigs, thyme and oregano
- 3 garlic cloves, peeled
- ½ lemon, cut into slices
- 1 tsp extra virgin olive oil
- Grinding of Himalayan salt and pepper

Preparation

1. Pre-heat the oven to 375 F.
2. Spatchcock the whole chicken as described above.
3. Place chicken in a large heavy oven-safe skillet.
4. Tuck fresh herbs, garlic cloves, lemon slices beneath the Spatchcocked chicken.
5. Brush with olive oil and season with a grinding of salt & pepper.
6. Place on the middle rack of the pre-heated oven and bake until the internal temperature of the chicken reaches 165 F (test both white and dark meat areas). Slice and serve.

Yield: 4 servings

Nutritional Information:

- Total Calories/serving: 278
- Total Carbs: 1 g
- Fiber: 0 g
- Total Fat: 7 g
- Protein: 24 g

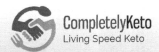

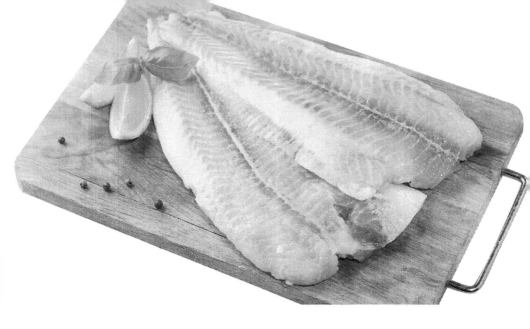

Fish Fry

Into the pan and onto a plate in minutes! Here's a quick meal for a busy family.

Ingredients

- 2 lb boneless Haddock fillets
- 2 T ghee
- Grinding of pink Himalayan salt & black pepper
- ½ tsp thyme leaves

Preparation

1. Melt ghee in a heavy bottomed skillet over medium high heat
2. Pat fillets dry, season both sides with salt & pepper and sprinkle the thyme on the top side.
3. Place fillets in pre-heated pan leaving a bit of room around each fillet and fry for 3 minutes on each side. Serve immediately while still hot.

Yield: 4 servings

Nutritional Information:

- Total Calories/serving: 271
- Total Carbs: 0 g
- Fiber: 0 g
- Total Fat: 10 g
- Protein: 43 g

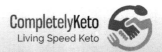

CompletelyKeto
Living Speed Keto

Veggies & Sides

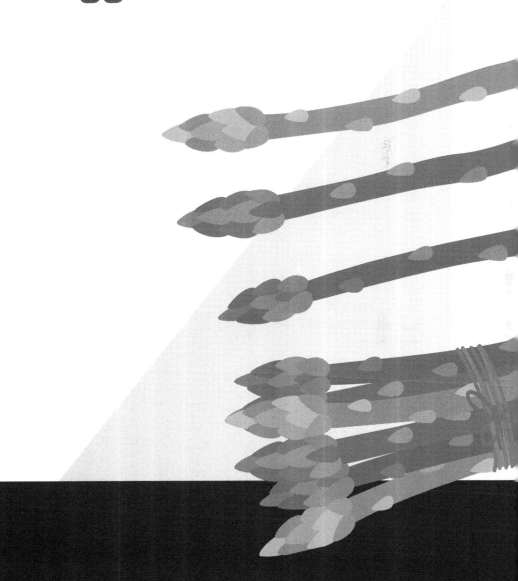

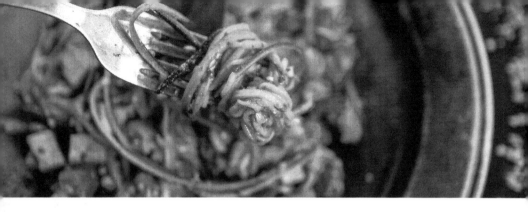

Zucchini "Noodles"

Served under your favorite keto sauce or as a side-dish, these zucchini noodles are a tasty alternative to traditional pasta. You can make the noodles by hand or, even easier, use a spiralizer!

Ingredients

- 2 small zucchini
- 2 T extra virgin olive oil
- 1 garlic clove, minced or pushed through a press

Preparation

1. To make the "noodles": Use a vegetable peeler to make long thin vertical slices along the side of one of the zucchini. Continue to peel thin slices until you reach the soft seeded core of the zucchini. Rotate the zucchini and repeat the process. Continue doing this until you've worked your way around the whole zucchini and discard the core. Repeat with the second zucchini. Alternatively you can simply use a vegetable spiralizer (if you are lucky enough to have one!).

2. Heat the olive oil in a heavy bottomed skillet over medium high heat and add the prepared zucchini "noodles" and minced garlic. Stir-fry the noodles for 3 or 4 minutes until the zucchini softens but is not over-cooked and mushy.

Yield: Serves 2

Nutritional Information:

- Total Calories/serving: 151
- Total Carbs: 7 g
- Fiber: 2 g
- Total Fat: 14 g
- Protein: 1 g

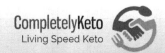

CompletelyKeto
Living Speed Keto

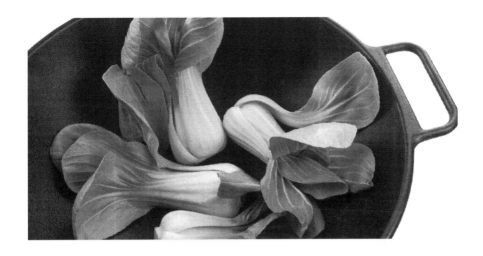

Baby Bok Choy Stir-fry

Add something exotic to your menu and stir-frying some chopped baby bok choy. This side-dish cooks up quickly and the garlic/ginger flavors will add some extra flavor to your meal. Left-over chicken, pork or beef turn this side into a meal in one bowl!

Ingredients

- 1 T extra virgin olive oil or ghee
- 2 garlic cloves
- 1" piece of fresh ginger, minced
- 8 C chopped baby bok choy
- 2 T wheat-free tamari sauce
- Grinding of pink Himalayan salt & pepper, to taste

Preparation

1. Heat oil in a wok (or heavy bottomed, deep skillet) over medium high heat.

2. Add remaining ingredients and stir-fry for 4 or 5 minutes. Serve immediately.

Yield: Serves 4

Nutritional Information:

- Total Calories/serving: 85
- Total Carbs: 7 g
- Fiber: 2 g
- Total Fat: 6 g
- Protein: 3 g

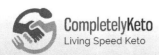
CompletelyKeto
Living Speed Keto

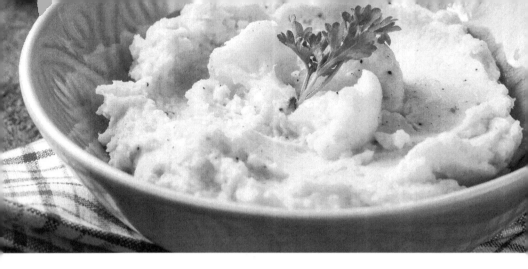

Cauliflower Mash with Roasted Garlic

For creamy cauliflower mash you will need to take care when squeezing the excess moisture out of the steamed cauliflower. It's a bit of a messy process but the end result is worth your effort. The mash will be creamier and thicker ... just the way you like it!

Ingredients

- 1 ½ heads of cauliflower, cut into florets
- 1 garlic bulb
- 3 T ghee, melted
- ¼ tsp pink Himalayan salt flakes
- ¼ tsp black pepper

Preparation

1. Pre-heat oven to 375 F.

2. Remove excess paper from garlic bulb and brush off any loose dirt from the root end. Use a sharp knife to cut off a bit of the top part of the bulb but leave the root end intact. Place bulb on a baking sheet and onto the middle rack of the pre-heated oven. Bake for 25 minutes or until the bulb turns a golden brown and the individual cloves inside the bulb are soft. When cool enough to handle, separate the cloves and remove the papery coating. Chop roughly into smaller chunks and set aside.

3. Steam cauliflower over boiling water until very tender. Transfer cooked cauliflower to a deep bowl.

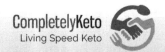

CompletelyKeto
Living Speed Keto

4. Using paper towel squeeze as much excess moisture as possible out of the flowerets by pressing down on them. The moisture will wick up into the paper towel. Don't worry if the cauliflower falls apart during this process.

5. Add the melted ghee and chopped garlic. Mash the cauliflower using a hand-held blender. Don't be afraid that the mash will get gluey by over-processing. It's the starch in potatoes that does that and since there's no starch in cauliflower you don't have to worry!

6. Correct the seasoning with salt and pepper. Serve while hot.

Serves 6

Nutritional Information:

- Total Calories/serving: 98
- Total Carbs: 8 g
- Fiber: 4 g
- Net Carbs: 4 g
- Total Fat: 7 g
- Protein: 3 g

Cauliflower Hash Browns

Cauliflower hash browns are a versatile side-dish at home next to turkey bacon and eggs in the morning and equally satisfying when served next to a beef roast at dinner time.

Ingredients

- 3 cups grated cauliflower (about one medium sized head)
- 2 T cooking onion, minced
- 1 egg
- 2 garlic cloves, minced or pushed through a press
- 1/2 tsp Himalayan salt
- ¼ tsp pepper
- 2 T ghee

Preparation

1. Use a box grater or food processor to grate cauliflower; 3 cups altogether.

2. Microwave for 4 minutes and let cool. Squeeze out any excess moisture. I use folded over paper towel placed overtop, and then

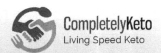

CompletelyKeto
Living Speed Keto

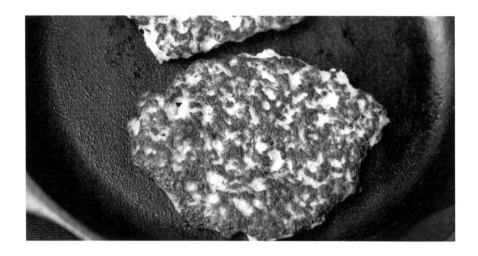

Cauliflower Hash Browns (continued)

press down on the micro-waved cauliflower using a flat-bottomed mug. This wicks the moisture up into the paper towel.

3. Add the remaining ingredients and combine.

4. Stove-top method: Melt half of the ghee in a heavy bottomed skillet over medium high heat. Make three mounds of the hash brown mixture in the hot pan and flatten each mound into an oval shape. Fry for 2 or 3 minutes then flip and continue cooking until the hash brown is crispy and cooked through. Repeat with the remaining batter making 6 hash browns in all.

5. Oven method: Form into six oval shaped hash browns on a parchment lined rimmed baking sheet.

6. Place on the middle rack of the pre-heated oven (400F) for 15-20 minutes.

7. Let cool for 10 minutes and they will firm up.

Yield: 6 hash browns (1 hash brown per serving)

Nutritional Information:

- Total Calories/serving: 84
- Total Carbs: 6 g
- Fiber: 3 g
- Total Fat: 6 g
- Protein: 3 g

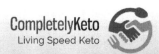

CompletelyKeto
Living Speed Keto

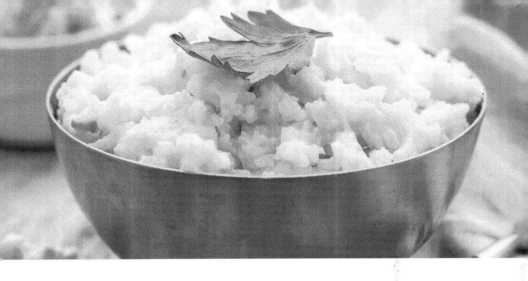

Cauliflower "Rice"

You can use a variety of different spices and herbs to create different flavor profiles for this tasty "rice". It's a versatile side-dish that works well with many different entrées.

Ingredients

- 2 T extra virgin olive oil or coconut oil
- 2 C cauliflower, grated
- ¼ C onion, fine dice
- 2 garlic cloves, minced

Preparation

- Melt ghee in a wok or heavy skillet over medium/high heat.
- Sauté onion for 3 minutes or until soft.
- Add minced garlic and sauté for one more minute.
- Add grated cauliflower and stir-fry for about 4 or 5 minutes until the rice is soft and cooked through. Remove from heat and serve immediately.

Yield: 4 servings (1/2 C each)

Nutritional Information:

- Total Calories/serving: 86
- Total Carbs: 4 g
- Fiber: 1 g
- Total Fat: 8 g
- Protein: 1 g

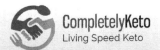

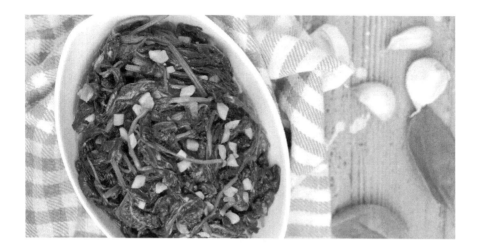

Spinach & Garlic Side Dish

Here's a recipe for a quick and easy side that I make often!

Ingredients

- 2 tsp extra virgin oil
- 4 garlic cloves, minced
- 8 C baby spinach leaves
- Squeeze of fresh lemon juice, if desired

Preparation

1. Heat oil in a heavy bottomed skillet over medium high heat. Add minced garlic and sauté for 1 minute.
2. Add half of the spinach and stir while spinach wilts before adding the remaining spinach to the skillet. Continue to sauté for 3 minutes or until the spinach is cooked to your liking.
3. Correct the seasoning with salt and pepper and serve with a quick squeeze of lemon over-top if desired.

Yield: serves 6

Nutritional Information:

- Total Calories/serving: 26
- Total Carbs: 1 g
- Fiber: 0 g
- Total Fat: 3 g
- Protein: 0 g

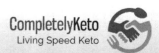

CompletelyKeto
Living Speed Keto

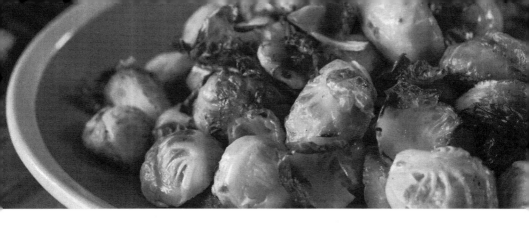

Roasted Brussels Sprouts

Roasting deepens the flavor of Brussels sprouts transforming them into sweet and salty morsels of pure pleasure. This is my favorite way to prepare Brussels sprouts. The preparation takes only minutes making this veggie side dish an easy choice.

Ingredients

- 1 lb Brussels sprouts
- 2 T extra virgin olive oil
- ½ tsp pink Himalayan salt
- ¼ tsp freshly ground black pepper

Preparation

1. Pre-heat the oven to 375 F.
2. Place Brussels sprouts in large bowl
3. Drizzle olive oil over-top and sprinkle on the salt and pepper. Toss until evenly coated with oil, salt and pepper
4. Turn out onto non-stick rimmed baking sheet and distribute evenly across the pan.
5. Place on the middle rack of the pre-heated oven. Bake for 35-45 minutes (depending on size of Brussels sprouts). Give the pan a shake every 10 minutes to ensure the Brussels sprouts brown evenly as they roast.
6. Serve immediately.

Yield: 4 servings

Nutritional Information:

- Total Calories/serving: 108
- Total Carbs: 10 g
- Fiber: 5 g
- Total Fat: 7 g
- Protein: 4 g

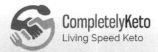

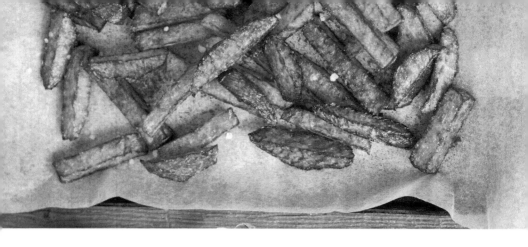

Turnip "Fries"

Pair these fries with just about anything! They add appeal to most any meals and will curb any fries-type cravings you may be having

Ingredients

- 4 turnips, cut into fries
- 2 T coconut oil
- Grinding of pink Himalayan salt & black pepper
- ½ tsp garlic powder
- Cayenne, to taste if desired

Preparation

1. Pre-heat oven to 425 F
2. Melt coconut oil and toss with turnip. Place turnip on a foil lined rimmed baking sheet. Leave space around the fries so they brown nicely.
3. Grind salt & pepper over-top. Sprinkle on the garlic powder and cayenne (if using). Place on the middle rack of the pre-heated oven and bake for 25 minutes.
4. Flip fries and bake for 20 more minutes or until golden brown and done.

Yield: 4 servings

Nutritional Information:

- Total Calories/serving: 79
- Total Carbs: 7 g
- Fiber:4 g
- Total Fat: 1 g
- Protein: 1 g

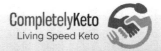

CompletelyKeto
Living Speed Keto

Salads & Dressings

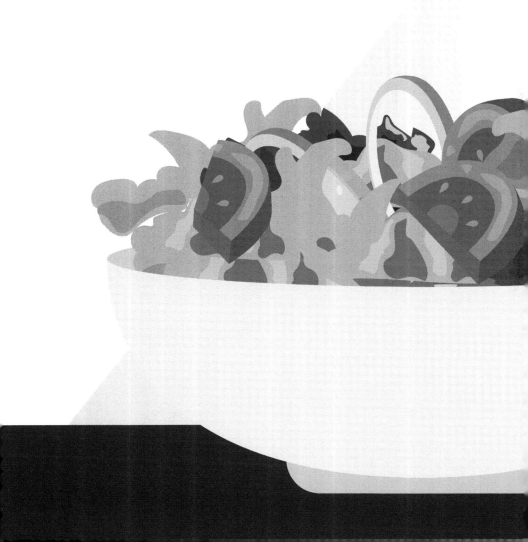

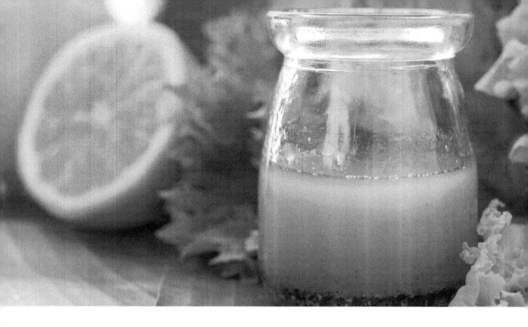

Vinaigrette

Homemade vinaigrettes are easy to make. Once you get onto how easy it is to whip one up there will be no going back to heavy handed, fake tasting store bought salad dressings.

Ingredients

- Juice from 1 lemon or 2 limes
- 1 tsp Dijon mustard
- 3 drops of liquid stevia
- ¾ C olive oil

Preparation

1. Whisk lemon juice, mustard and liquid stevia.

2. Drizzle olive oil into the lemon juice mixture and continue whisking until all the oil has been incorporated into the dressing.

Yield: 16 servings (1 Tablespoon in each serving)

Nutritional Information:

- Total Calories/serving: 90
- Total Carbs: 0 g
- Fiber: 0 g
- Total Fat: 10 g
- Protein: 0 g

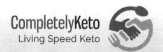

CompletelyKeto
Living Speed Keto

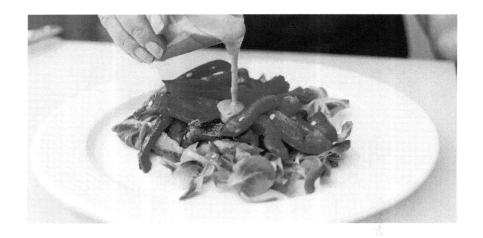

Completely Keto Green Goddess Dressing

This dressing was invented and served to me by a friend. I begged for the recipe. Use this dressing for a change on any of the salads we have listed on the menu.

Ingredients

- 2 ripe avocados, peeled and stone removed
- 2 garlic cloves, minced or pushed through a press
- ½ C green onions (scallions), chopped
- 1 ½ T fresh dill, chopped
- ¼ C parsley, chopped
- 1 T fresh lemon juice
- ½ T fresh lime juice
- 1 ½ T extra virgin olive oil
- Freshly ground pink Himalayan salt & black pepper, to taste

Preparation

1. Put all ingredients in food processor and process until creamy.

Yield: 4 servings

Nutritional Information:

- Total Calories/serving: 161
- Total Carbs: 9 g
- Fiber: 6 g
- Net Carbs: 3 g
- Total Fat: 14 g

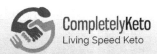

CompletelyKeto
Living Speed Keto

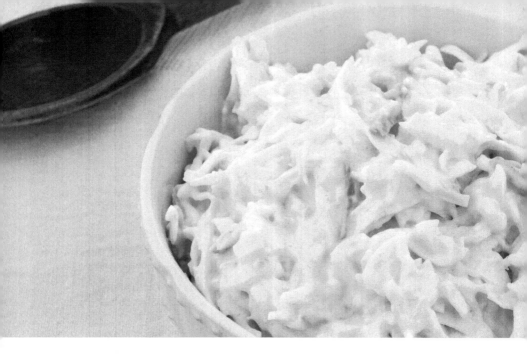

Keto Coleslaw

Coleslaw; a salad that's stood the test of time. We've tweaked the recipe to make it keto friendly, so dig in and enjoy!

Ingredients

- 3 C shredded cabbage
- 1 dill pickle, small dice
- 3 T onion, minced
- 3 T mayonnaise
- ½ T pickle juice
- Salt and pepper to taste

Preparation

1. Mix all ingredients together and serve.

Yield: 4 servings (reserve one portion for lunch tomorrow)

Nutritional Information:

- Total Calories/serving: 91
- Total Carbs: 5 g
- Fiber: 2 g
- Total Fat: 8 g
- Protein: 1 g

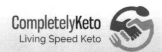

CompletelyKeto
Living Speed Keto

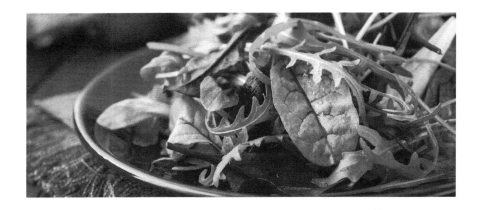

Every Day Green Salad

Ingredients

- 2 C mixed greens of your choice
- 2 C baby spinach leaves
- 2 green onions (scallions), thinly sliced
- ¼ C English cucumber, small dice
- ½ avocado, sliced (if desired)
- 2 T vinaigrette (see recipe), or other allowed dressing of choice

Preparation

1. Toss mixed greens, spinach, cucumber and green onions together in a salad bowl
2. Drizzle vinaigrette over-top.
3. Toss and serve immediately.

Yield: Serves 4

Nutritional Information:
(without avocado)

- Total Calories/serving: 193
- Total Carbs: 6 g
- Fiber: 4 g
- Total Fat: 19 g
- Protein: 2 g

Nutritional Information:
(with avocado)

- Total Calories/serving: 307
- Total Carbs: 12 g
- Fiber: 9 g
- Total Fat: 30 g
- Protein: 3 g

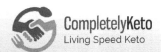

CompletelyKeto
Living Speed Keto

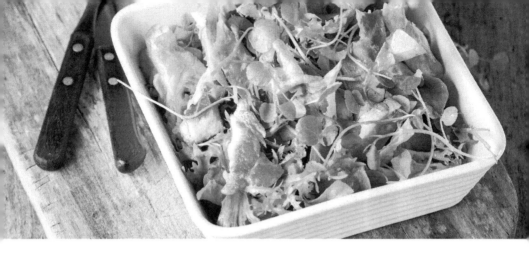

Easy Caesar Salad for Two

A Caesar Salad on the side dresses up a meal nicely. Add left-over chicken and you have a perfect meal in one bowl for lunch or dinner. Sprinkle on some crumbled cooked bacon for a change every once in awhile.

Ingredients

- 1 ½ C romaine lettuce, torn into pieces
- ½ C arugula
- 1 clove garlic, finely minced.
- ½ tsp anchovy paste (optional)
- ¼ tsp Worcestershire sauce.
- 2 tsp fresh lemon juice
- ½ tsp Dijon mustard.
- ¼ C full fat mayonnaise.
- Salt & Pepper to taste.

Preparation

1. Place torn romaine leaves into salad bowl.
2. In a separate bowl whisk anchovy paste, Worcestershire sauce, lemon juice, Dijon mustard and mayonnaise. Add salt & pepper to taste. Drizzle salad dressing over the romaine, toss & serve.

Yield: Serves 2

Nutritional Information:

- Total Calories/serving: 194
- Total Carbs: 2 g
- Fiber: 1 g
- Total Fat: 20 g
- Protein: 1 g

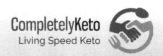

CompletelyKeto
Living Speed Keto

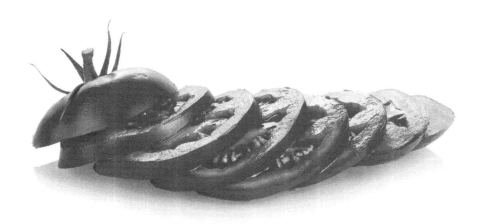

Plattered Tomato Salad

Ingredients

- 2 large tomatoes, sliced
- 6 Mediterranean style black olives, pitted and chopped
- 1 thin slice red onion, rings pulled apart
- 1 T capers
- ¼ C Vinaigrette

Preparation

1. Fan out tomato slices on a platter and sprinkle the onion rings, black olive and capers over-top evenly.

2. Drizzle on the Vinaigrette. If you make this salad about ½ hour ahead of serving time the flavors will meld nicely.

Yield: Serves 4

Nutritional Information:

- Total Calories/serving: 123
- Total Carbs: 3 g
- Fiber: 1 g
- Total Fat: 12 g
- Protein: 1 g

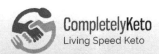

CompletelyKeto
Living Speed Keto

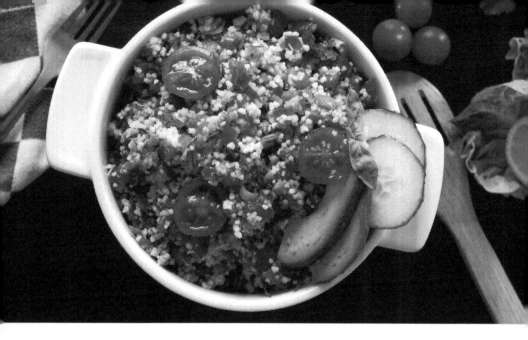

Harlan's Israeli Salad

I use cauliflower "rice" in place of couscous for this keto version of a traditional Israeli salad. I also roast the tomatoes and garlic to deepen their flavors and bring out the natural sweetness but you can skip this step if pressed for time.

Ingredients

- ½ C cauliflower "rice" (use ¾ C florets to make "rice")
- ½ C red cherry tomatoes, cut in half
- 2 garlic cloves
- 1 tsp dried oregano (or 1 T fresh, minced)
- Juice of one lemon
- 2 T extra virgin olive oil
- ¼ C pitted Mediterranean style black olives, chopped
- ¼ C red onion, small dice
- ¼ C English cucumber, small dice
- ¼ C flat leaf parsley, roughly chopped
- ¼ C fresh mint leaved, roughly chopped
- Salt & pepper, to taste

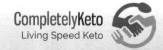

CompletelyKeto
Living Speed Keto

Harlan's Israeli Salad (continued)

Preparation

1. Pre-heat oven to 350°F.
2. Make cauliflower rice by using a food processor or grate by hand. Place the "rice" in a microwavable glass dish and cover with plastic wrap, leaving a small gap for steam to escape. Microwave on high setting until the cauliflower bits are softened but not mushy. Time will vary depending on the wattage of your microwave. Allow the cauliflower rice to cool and refrigerate until ready to assemble the salad.
3. Cut tomatoes in half and arrange on a parchment lined baking sheet. Add garlic cloves to pan and drizzle 1 tablespoon of the olive oil over-top. Roast on the middle rack of the pre-heated oven until tomatoes are slightly charred and the garlic cloves are softened. This should take 25-30 minutes. Cool in pan for 30 before handling.
4. To make a dressing, remove outer skin from the garlic cloves and place in a blender with ¼ C of the roasted tomatoes. Add the dried oregano, lemon juice and olive oil. Process on high, until tomatoes and garlic become completely blended with the oil and lemon juice.
5. When everything has cooled toss together the cauliflower "rice", remaining roasted tomatoes, black olives, cucumbers, red onion, parsley and mint. Add the dressing, toss again and serve.

Yield: serves 2

Nutritional Information:

- Total Calories/serving: 177
- Total Carbs: 10 g
- Fiber: 2 g
- Total Fat: 15 g
- Protein: 2 g

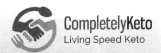

CompletelyKeto
Living Speed Keto

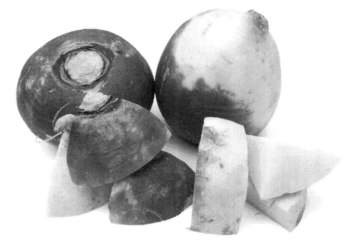

Mock Potato Salad

It may seem strange to substitute turnip for potatoes but we urge you to give it a try. The flavor of this mock potato salad comes pretty close to the original. It won't disappoint!

Ingredients

- 3 C cubed raw turnip
- 3 eggs, hard cooked
- ¼ C green onion, thin slices
- ½ C mayonnaise
- Grinding of pink Himalayan salt and black pepper, to taste

Preparation

1. Boil turnip until it softens but isn't mushy. Drain, cool then refrigerate
2. Boil eggs until hard (about 15 minutes for eggs that come straight from the fridge). Cool, then refrigerate.
3. When you are ready to make your salad, peel eggs and mash with a fork in a in a medium sized bowl.
4. Add cooked turnip, green onion slices and mayonnaise. Mix well and season with salt & pepper, to taste. Garnish with a sprinkle of paprika before serving.

Yield: serves 6

Nutritional Information:

- Total Calories/serving: 134
- Total Carbs: 4 g
- Fiber: 1 g
- Total Fat: 12 g
- Protein: 3 g

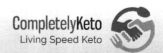

CompletelyKeto
Living Speed Keto

From Our Collection

If you like the information in this book, you may also enjoy these from our collection:

Keto Success Secrets Book

Everything you ever wanted to know about Keto, including how it works, why it works, how to get started, what to eat and how to fit Keto into your busy life.

Keto Success Secrets Quick Start Guide

Get started with Keto right away by following these five super-simple yet super-effective steps.

Keto On The Go Guide

Stay Keto when eating in restaurants, celebrating with friends, or grabbing some fast food with our Keto On The Go Guide.

Keto Success Secrets Shopping List

Save time and money by using our comprehensive shopping list to stock up on Keto foods. Get the ingredients to make delicious, satisfying meals and snacks so you never go hungry.

50 Easy Keto Recipes Book

I've handpicked the most delicious and easiest recipes, so you'll look forward to each and every meal without having to slave in the kitchen.

CompletelyKeto Cookbook

Treat yourself to delicious, comforting completely Keto food that actually help you burn fat faster. Includes Keto versions of all your favorites, like ribs, cheesecake, pretzels and cookies.

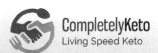

CompletelyKeto
Living Speed Keto

Cheesecake Cookbook

Our Completely Keto cheesecake recipe is one of the most searched and pinned on the planet. Get that recipe and 24 others, including Salted Caramel, Pumpkin, and White Chocolate Cheesecake in this limited edition.

Keto Recipe Collections

Never have to worry what to eat on your Keto way of life with our mouthwatering breakfast, lunch, dinner and dessert recipe collections. These trusted recipes are quick and easy to make too.

CompletelyKeto Electrolytes Formula

No need to suffer from Keto flu when you take our specially formulated electrolytes. These tasty, sugar-free drinks will keep you body hydrated and balanced as you burn the fat.

CompletelyKeto MCT Oil in Powder Form

Our MCT powder is nutritionally just like MCT oil but converted into a solid (powder) form that makes it easy to incorporate into baked foods and drinks and much softer on your digestive system.

Ketosis Training Institute

Become a Keto Coach and help others take control of their health, reach their ideal body and live their best lives. If you want to work flexible hours from home, this could be for you. Join here: www.CompletelyKeto.com/ktigroup

Questions? Our happy support team is here for you:

https://CompletelyKeto.com/support

CompletelyKeto
Living Speed Keto

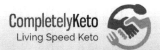

Index: Recipes A-Z

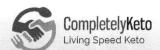

CompletelyKeto
Living Speed Keto

L

Lamb Souvlaki 26, 34, 50, 98

M

Mocha Smoothie 21, 28, 31, 35, 50, 62

Mock Potato Salad 28, 50, 100, 124

O

Old fashioned Chicken Noodle Soup 50

Oven Baked Baby Back Ribs 50, 100, 101

P

Perfectly Boiled Eggs 21, 31, 50, 61

Perfectly Poached Eggs 50, 58, 59, 64

Perfect Steak 24, 50, 91, 92

Plattered Tomato Salad 24, 30, 50, 121

Poached Egg with Hollandaise on Asparagus 23, 36, 50, 64

R

Roasted Brussels Sprouts 36, 50, 113

Roasted Spatchcocked Chicken 50, 103

Roasted Turkey Breast 22, 35, 50, 86

S

Seared Scallops on Sautéed Asparagus 50, 96

Simple Caesar Salad for Two 50

Simple Roast Chicken 21, 36, 50, 84, 85

Smokey BBQ Sauce 50

Spaghetti Bolognese 21, 34, 50, 82, 83

Speedy Fish Fry 50

Spinach Salad with Chicken 22, 32, 50, 74

Steamed Cauliflower & Broccoli 21, 50

Stir-fried Pork & Broccoli 50, 81

T

Tex/Mex Fish Roll-ups 29, 50, 102

Tuna Salad on Romaine (with Sliced Cucumber & Olives) 50

Turkey Buddha Lunch Bowl 23, 35, 50, 75

Turnip "Fries" 32, 50, 114

V

Vinaigrette 23, 35, 50, 75, 116, 121

Z

Zucchini "Noodles" 50, 106

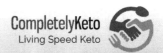

CompletelyKeto
Living Speed Keto